VOLCANO
ORDEAL BY FIRE
IN ICELAND'S
WESTMANN ISLANDS

VOLCANO

ORDEAL BY FIRE IN ICELAND'S WESTMANN ISLANDS

Iceland Review Books

Toil and Prosperity

Surtsey — the Omen and the Lesson

Off the southern coast of Iceland lies a cluster of islands by the name of Westman Islands or Vestmannaeyjar (eyjar=islands), as they will henceforth be called. One of the country's best-know poets has described these islands as sapphires set in a silver ring, and there is no doubt that here, in a relatively small area, may be found natural beauty that will not be surpassed elsewhere in Iceland. Majestic landscape, striking colours, and varied bird life all contribute to the splendour. The group consists of 15 islands, besides which there are some 55 or 60 known submarine craters. It lies at the southern end of the so-called eastern volcanic zone, which crosses Iceland from Melrakkaslétta in the north, through Mývatn, Askja, and Grímsvötn all the way south to Vestmannaeyjar, where it terminates. The western volanic zone running through Reykjanes, on the other hand, joins the Mid-Atlantic Ridge, which stretches south the entire length of the Atlantic.

On November 14, 1963, a submarine eruption began a short distance off the main cluster, southwest of an islet named Geirfuglasker. Residents of Heimaey, the largest of the islands and the only inhabited one, were able to follow closely the course of this eruption. It started at a depth of 130 metres, and during the first four months some 400 million cubic metres — about 40 cubic metres per second — of volcanic materials were discharged. At first, the sea broke down the new land as soon as it emerged above the surface. Two islands formed by the eruption vanished that way, and for a long time it was believed that the sea would finally triumph. One island, however, did endure — Surtsey. Here, a lava flow began in April, 1964, securing the island's future; the sea could not do away with the lava. Out of the ocean rose a virgin land, untouched but ready to receive whatever life might be carried there. Since then, this island has been a most remarkable research station, where scientists from many parts of the world have come to witness how life takes hold on a new piece of land. They have studied bird life, primal vegetation, algae in the surrounding waters, insect life, and other subjects, thereby gaining answers to some questions that were hitherto unsettled. Surtsey is the southernmost member of Vestmannaeyjar, and the eruption there provided first-hand knowledge of how the other islands in the group, including Heimaey, were formed. It is considered certain that most of them were created by submarine eruptions after the end of the last ice age, some 10,000—15,000 years ago.

While the sea had access to the volcanic vent of Surtsey, the eruption there was a so-called pyroclastic one, in which the ejected materials were pumice and ashes. But when the island had grown large enough to keep the sea away from the crater, lava began to flow. In time, the pumice and ashes usually become solid rock, called tuff (móberg), but before

Vestmannaeyjar are located a sho[rt] distance south of the Icelandic mainlan[d]. They rise, graceful and majestic, fro[m] the level of the sea. Around them a[re] some of the richest fishing banks [of] Icelan[d]

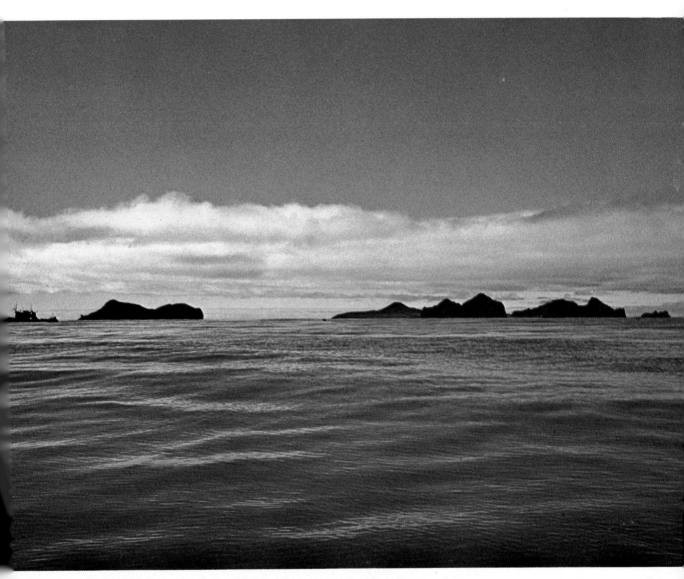

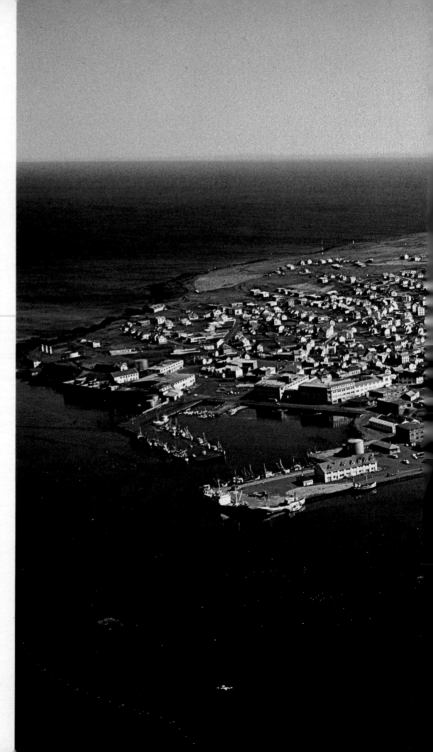

that could happen on Surtsey the sea broke down a large part of it. The same holds true for the formation of all the other islands. When lava begins to flow, however, it provides a new-born island with effective protection against the destructive force of the sea.

Most of the islands in the Vestmanna group are made of tuff, which has been shaped into perpendicular cliffs. Only on Heimaey, Ellidaey, and Bjarnarey was there a flow of lava. Heimaey is actually formed by the union, during eruptions, of two or more islands. A volcanic outburst of Helgafell on Heimaey some 5,000—6,000 years ago thus joined together two islets and at the same time fashioned the elegant cone of the volcano. Helgafell is one of the main features of the islands, and the town on Heimaey is built upon lava from the mountain. The islands of Ellidaey and Bjarnarey were created in a similar way at the same approximate time.

There are certainly not many places in the world where the inhabitants have been able to observe as closely as have the people of Vestmannaeyjar how their land was originally created. For nearly four years they could follow the course of the Surtsey eruption, watching how the island grew from day to day and, later, how life developed; such wonders do not happen frequently. They also witnessed how the awesome power of the sea transformed new land into an old in a short time, how the newly run lava became an old coast in a matter of days, and how the shape of the island was con-

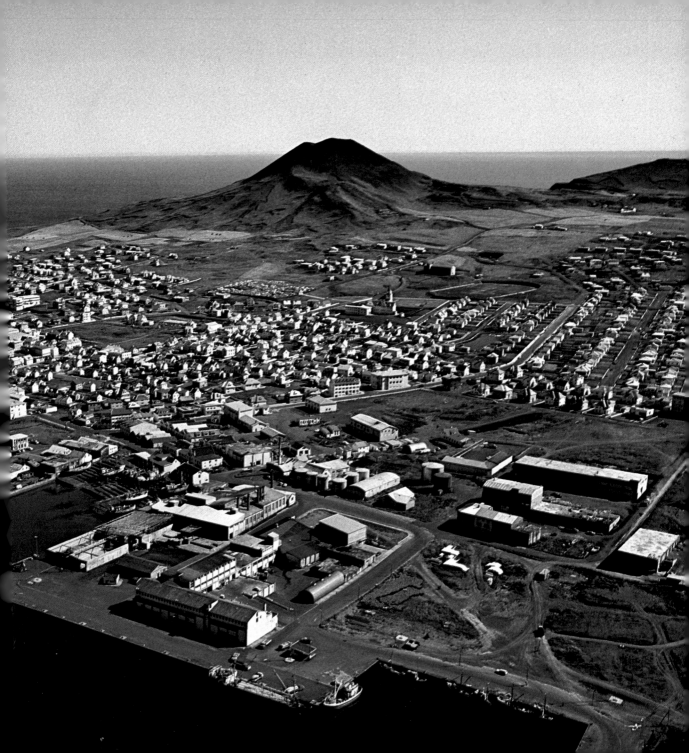

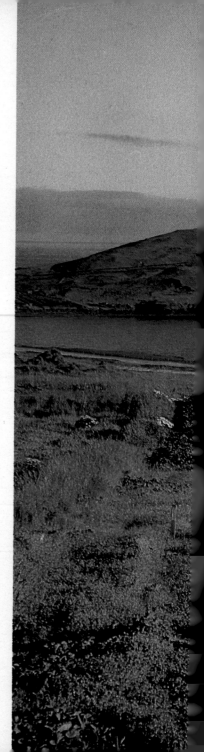

stantly changing. In the evening, when darkness began to fall, the fire in the vents became visible, as did the bolts of lightning in the cloud of smoke and vapour rising from the craters, and the glow from the streaming lava. Many made the trip out to the new island to walk about the land where, before, there had been fishing banks. The eruption became part of people's daily life; all they had to do was look out of their windows on Heimaey, and they would know how it was coming along. Finally, they even ceased to notice it.

To some, however, the quiet thought occurred that all this could just as well have happened on Heimaey, in the handsome little town standing on the lava from a volcano active 5,000—6,000 years ago. In Iceland, one of the most volcanic spots in the world, many people think that way. But no one will resign himself to the idea that his home may become the site of such a fiery outburst. At least, no one cares to pursue the thought to its conclusion.

A Look Back at History

How did Vestmannaeyjar appear to the people who first arrived there to settle? As seen from the mainland, the islands rise high above the sea, and in the mirage of a hot, sunny day they look still higher and closer to the coast. On approaching them, one is likely to notice first how precipitous they are and, second, how lush is the green colour that covers them from the top to the brink of their vertical cliff walls. Below that,

little or no vegetation can secure a foothold, and the colour is grayish or pure white; here, for centuries, thousands of birds have made their home. There is hardly any lowland on any of the islands, except Heimaey, which is by far the largest of them 4.34 square miles. The highest spot on Heimaey is Heimaklettur, 896 feet, followed by the volcanic cone of Helgafell, which is 678 feet.

The oldest account of Vestmannaeyjar is not one of peaceful endeavour — of people who landed, established a settlement, and lived happily ever after. It is a story of slayings. The first settler of Iceland was a Norwegian named Ingólfur Arnarson. He had a sworn brother by the name of Hjörleifur Hródmarsson. Before journeying to Iceland, where the two intended to settle, Hjörleifur had gone on a Viking raid to Ireland and gathered a great deal of loot. He also captured and bonded ten Irishmen, whom he later took with him to Iceland. The two blood brothers landed on the southern shore, about a day's journey apart, and there made their camps for the winter. In the spring, Hjörleifur wanted to plow a field and sow some grain, and he put his Irish thralls to work. The thralls, however, had a different idea. They killed Hjörleifur and then departed the wintering site, taking with them the women of the household, as well as Hjörleifur's chattels, including a boat. The story has it that the thralls used the boat to make their way to the island they saw lying offshore to the southwest.

When Ingólfur discovered the killing of

6

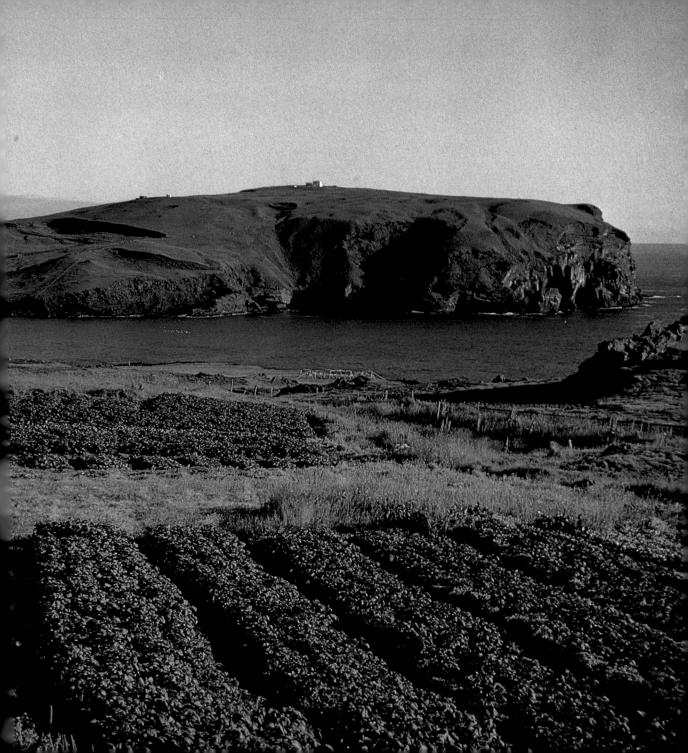

his sworn brother, he was bound by duty and custom to revenge him. Finding Hjörleifur's boat gone, he concluded that the thralls must have gone out to the islands and immediately pursued them with his retainers. Surprised while eating, the fearstricken thralls scattered, trying to get away, but were all run down and killed. Even to this day, there are place names in Vestmannaeyjar, which are said to be derived from the names of these thralls. What is more, according to the story, it was owing to this event that the islands acquired their name, meaning the Westmen's Islands; „Westmen" was the old Scandinavians' designation for Britons and Irishmen.

There are those who find it unlikely that Ingólfur could have killed all the thralls and believe that some of them may have survived and had offspring. Some scholars, skeptical of the story, have theorised that the islands were named for their first permanent settler, Herjólfur, who in all probability was a „Westman." But the story of Ingólfur is as good as any other. It is fairly certain that, while Ingólfur may have been there in 875, Vestmannaeyjar were not permanently settled until between 900 and 930. Before that, they were apparently used as a fishing station without wintering facilities. Until the 12th century, the islands were owned by he local farmers. Most of them were then bought by an Icelandic bishop, with the idea of establishing a monastery. That, however, never came to pass, but the islands were owned by the bishopric until the early 15th

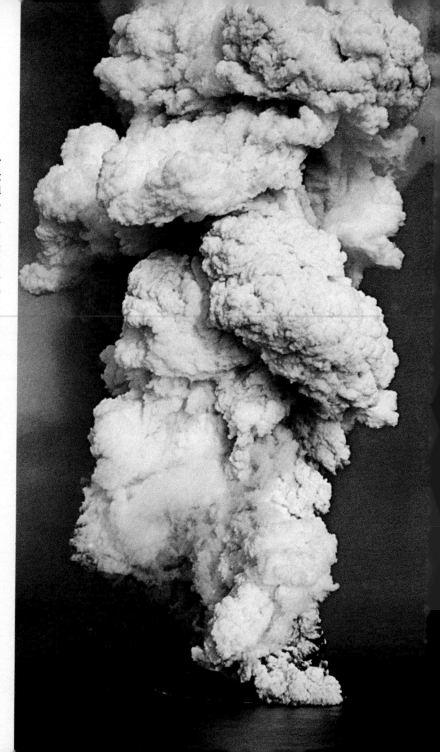

*For almost four years the people of
Vestmannaeyjar could follow an eruption, which
had its submarine origins on 14 November 1963.
This was a powerful eruption, and gradually a
new island rose from the sea, which was
eventually called Surtsey.*

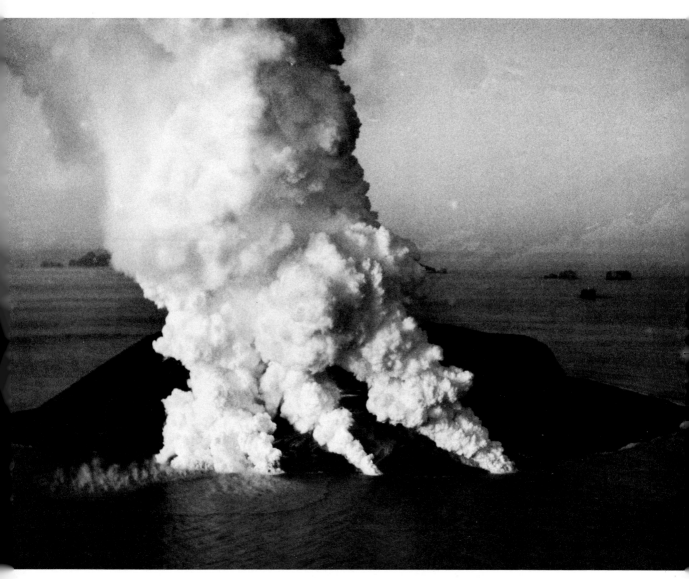

century. The story is that sometime after 1420 King Eric of Pomerania (who was then King of Denmark) acquired the islands as payment of a large debt owed him by an Icelandic bishop. Vestmannaeyjar remained the property of the Danish kings for a long time afterward. They are now owned by the Icelandic republic. Resident magistrates were first appointed to the islands around 1700, and in 1787 they were issued a town charter, but that charter was revoked in 1807. A new one was granted in 1918, at which time it was also decreed that there should be a bailiff and a town council.

There has been a church in Vestmannaeyjar ever since Christianity was adopted in Iceland in the year 1000.

Little is known about the population of the islands during the first centuries of settlement, except that many people seem to have moved there from the closest mainland districts. The first census, taken in 1703, showed the population to be 318. During the following decades, experience proved that when the fishing was good, the population increased, while it decreased again when times were harder. Around 1800 there were only 173 inhabitants; their number had been diminished due to small catches and hard times caused by volcanic eruptions on the mainland. After the turn of the 20th century, the population began to increase rapidly; it reached 3,347 in 1930, and by 1940 it exceeded 3,500. At the end of 1972 there were 5,273 people on the islands.

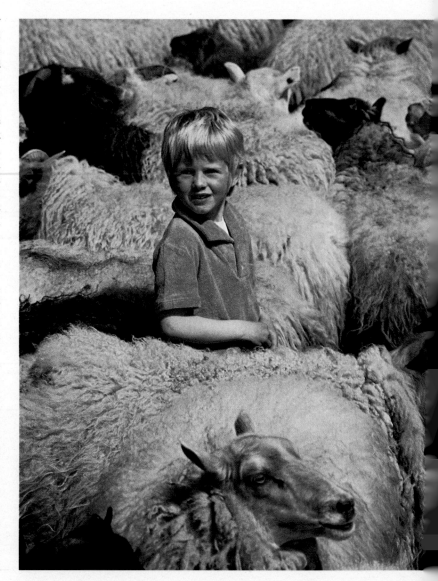

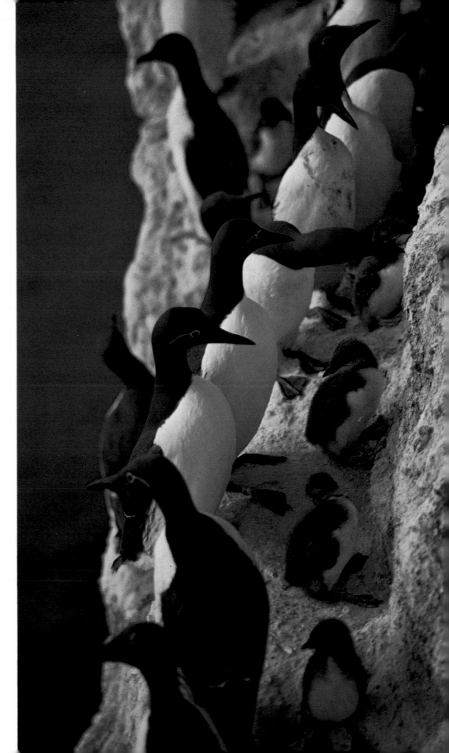

Life in Vestmannaeyjar is luxuriant. There were sheep and cattle in considerable numbers. And the bird life is flourishing, peaceful – but noisy. The birds are everywhere, in the cliffs and on the sea.

As evidenced by the fluctuations of the population, Vestmannaeyjar have known their share of hardships. From the earliest times, the people have depended on fishing for their livelihood, and there has also been much bird catching. The fisheries have cost unnumbered lives, but the islanders are considered among the hardiest and best fishermen in Iceland, although for centuries they themselves did not own any worthwhile fishing vessels. While Iceland was under Danish rule, the fisheries were all run by the royal monopoly and its licenced agents. The islanders manned the king's ships and those of his monopolist merchants, receiving little for their toil. Disasters were frequent, adding up to hundreds of drowned fishermen.

But the people of Vestmannaeyjar did not give up — not even when they were horribly struck by foreign marauders. In 1614 English freebooters raided the islands, plundering and looting, manhandling the people, and leaving with a large booty. Thirteen years later, in July, 1627, another band of pirates arrived at the islands in three ships. These pillagers have been traditionally called Turks, but actually they were of many nationalities and came from the city of Sla, which is now a part of Rabat, the capital of Morocco. Their leader was a Dutchman, one of the most infamous pirates of his time. He had raided the mainland a few days earlier, robbing and ravaging. People in Vestmannaeyjar were totally defenseless against their barbarism. It is estimated that the population at the time was about 500. The pirates killed 36 people, and kidnapped 242. They combed the islands in search of those who had hidden in caves and holes, and the captives were bound and put aboard the ships. Anyone who moved too slowly for the pirates, be it a child or a decrepit old woman, was hacked to pieces. Many old people were burned alive after their homes had been ransacked. The surviving captives were sold into slavery. It was a devastating blow to the small community.

Where Birds and People Prosper

The Vestmannaeyjar are surrounded by some of the richest fishing grounds in Icelandic waters, and the islands have long been one of the most important fishing harbours in the country. In some ways, they may be compared with the notorious „gold" towns of the United States, where prospectors gathered to make a fast buck. During the fishing seasons, young men and women flock to Vestmannaeyjar to work for a few months, and while the season lasts there is no more bustling place in all of Iceland.

As late as 1905, fishing was done only by rowboats, in which there was no shelter against the elements, and seamen had to rely on their own physical strength. But the fishing grounds were near, and the catches were good. In 1906, the first motorised fishing boats were brought to the islands; by 1929, there were 97 of them. The value of the catch increased steadily, and all kinds of dependent esta-

blishments were founded: icehouses, liver oil plants, netmaker shops, fish-meal factories, fish export firms, machine shops, shipyards, slipways, and various others. Then, like the rest of the western world, the Vestmannaeyjar were hit by the Depression, and many businesses went bankrupt after flourishing for thirty years. Nevertheless, people carried on, and few pulled in their oars altogether. World War II brought a sudden change for the better: „one man's meat is another man's poison." The nations of Europe needed fish, and there was plenty of it around Vestmannaeyjar. The whole economy revived. Processing plants were built, new boats with modern equipment were bought, and the catches became larger than ever before. The community on Heimaey grew steadily and so did its prosperity. Many energetic businessmen moved to the islands, founding profitable firms. Once more, the islands had recovered from a crippling blow.

Farming land in Vestmannaeyjar is very limited. Although the islands are, in places, very grassy, on the whole, the vegetation is scant and unvaried. There are no streams, brooks, or wetlands, and the lack of water has often been troublesome. Classified species of plants on the islands number about 120, and some 80 or 90 species of insects have been found. Because the land area is so limited, agriculture has always been on a very small scale. Although in a few years before 1930, improved farming methods more than doubled the hay harvest, the outer islands have had to be cropped in order

Abrupt cliffs, thousands of sea fowl sitting on eggs in the spring. A scene typical of Vestmannaeyjar where there is always bustling life

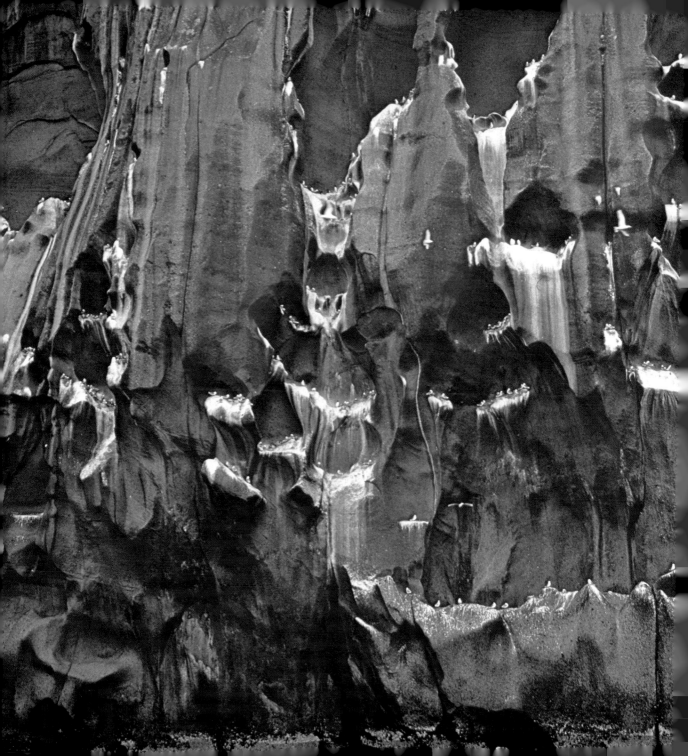

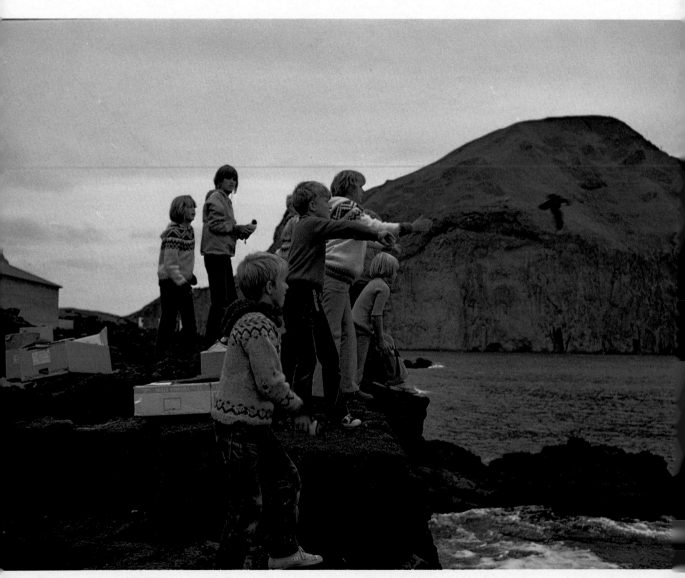

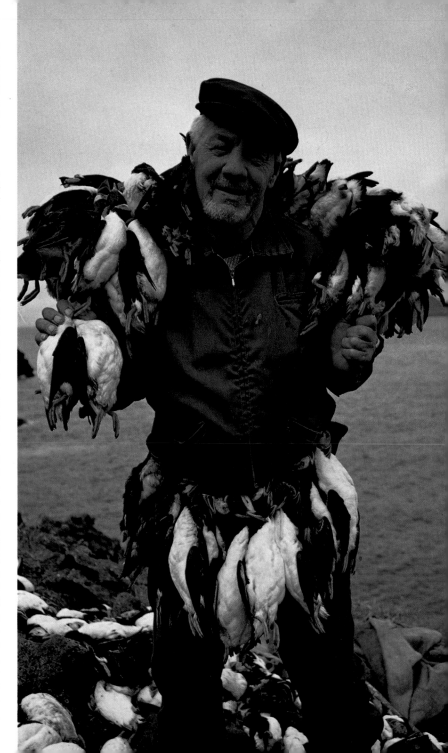

to make enough hay for the livestock. Cattle and sheep are traditionally the most numerous, but animal husbandry has been decreasing in recent years, especially after the town began to purchase milk from the mainland.

Few places in Iceland enjoy more varied bird life than Vestmannaeyjar, and the birds have left a definite mark on the environment and the aspect of the islands. There is a continuous sound of croaking from the bird cliffs, which reaches the ear like a gentle, even drone that never stops. The birds soar on winds and rising air currents along the cliffs, and one can watch them endlessly, following their flights in a never-ending search for food, abundant in the deep by the cliffs. They build their nests surprisingly close together and sometimes so precariously near the brink of ledges and crags that one would expect them to drop into the sea at the slightest hint of a wind. But there they sit, and the birds have inhabited the same cliffs for centuries on end. The puffin is the most numerous, but there are also immense numbers of razorbill, black guillemot, fulmar, and kittiwake. The queen of the sea, the gannet, colonizes the outer islands, and Leach's petrel, Manx shearwater, and gulls also nest there in a few places. In former times, egg-gathering and bird-catching was widely practiced in the islands, but today only a few hardy men go to the outer islands each summer to catch puffin. Then, for a period of four to five weeks in July and August, they stay in small cots teetering on the brinks

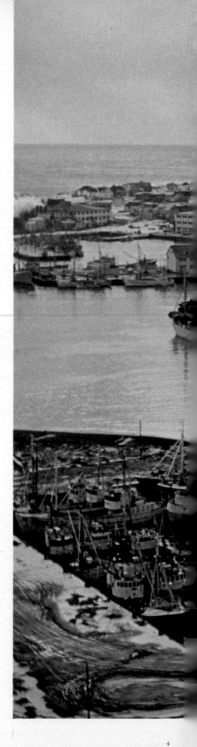

of the islands' precipices and lead the free life — eating when they feel hungry, sleeping when they get drowsy. At other times, they may be found in the puffin colonies, catching the birds in landing nets as they fly against the wind along the brink of the cliff walls. When a bird comes within reach, the fowler darts out his net, pulls in the bird, and wrings its neck. This goes on all day long, weather permitting. At the end of the day the birds are collected, tied up in bunches, and thrown over the cliff into the sea, where a boat will be waiting for the catch.

The puffin nests in holes, which it digs into the ground. It is a very gregarious bird, and the burrows are close together; the colonies can resemble big ant hills and are often difficult to walk through. A bird of passage, the puffin arrives in April and departs in the fall. A trained fowler may catch 300—400 birds a day. During the 19th century the puffin was netted for its feathers which were sold abroad. But the killing became excessive; in 1861 alone some 25,000 pounds of feathers were exported. Extermination could be foreseen, and netting was then prohibited. At that time, the gathering of fulmar chicks and eggs was also widely practiced. This was done by lowering someone over the face of the cliffs. A rope was attached to an experienced catcher, while six or seven others braced themselves on the brink and held the line, heaving or lowering according to indications from the fowler. It was a dangerous occupation and has been largely abandoned.

Whoever visits the bird colonies in Vestmannaeyjar will never forget the experience. Every spring he will be seized by a yearning to go back — to enjoy the outdoor life, the unspoiled nature, and the presence of the birds. The bird life is one of the most attractive elements of the islands' environment and the one that most impresses young and old alike, both natives and foreigners. This is particularly true of the young people of Heimaey, children and teenagers. In August, after the evenings begin to get dark again, they comb the piers and the streets of the town to save the puffin chicks, which, attracted by the street lights, have flown in from the cliffs sheltering the harbour. The parent birds, by that time, have abandoned their young, and when the chicks get hungry they drop over the cliffs in search of food, beating the air with their wings for the first time. They fly toward the lights in town, alight in the streets or on the quays and do not have the strength to take off again. The children pick up the birds, put them in a box, and at dawn the following day take them up to the cliffs and literally throw them up in the air, so that they may fly again and get by on their own.

Self-Reliant People

There can be no doubt about it that owing to their location, the Vestmannaeyjar have developed into one of the most remarkable communities in Iceland. The islanders have long had to

16

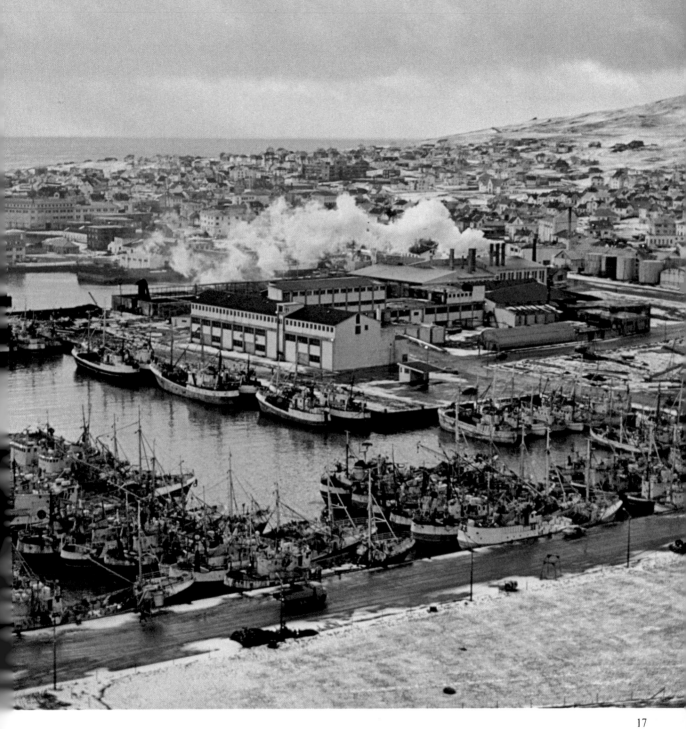

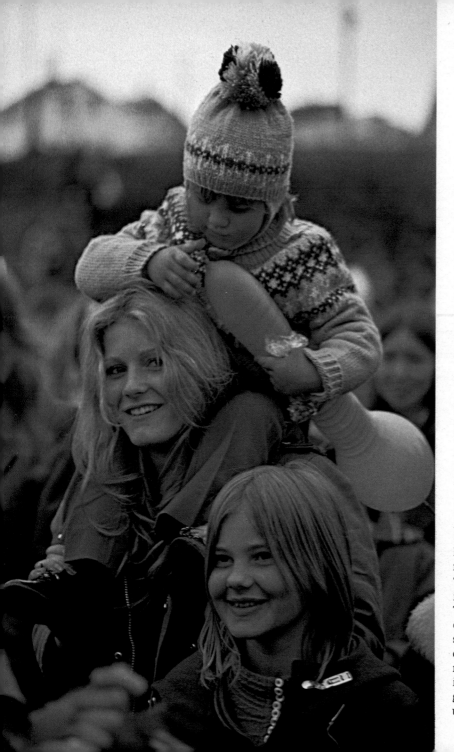

rely on their own strength and enter-
prise for all their needs. Time and again
they have suffered catastrophes, some of
which have already been mentioned, but it
has only made them tougher. An example
of their initiative is the establishment
in 1862 of the first Icelandic insurance
company. It is still in business. Its founding was due simply to the necessity created by the daily life of the people. The
sea, then as now, was the source of livelihood for a large number of the islanders, and many inevitably perished. In
1685, for instance, fifty seamen from
Vestmannaeyjar drowned on a single
day. In 1757, another fifty men were
lost at sea in one day. Widows and
children were left without a breadwinn-
er, which in most cases meant destitute.
Large-scale fisheries also required a good
harbour. The first breakwater was begun
in 1914. That one crumbled the following winter under the ceaseless pounding
by the storm-driven waves of the ocean.
But it was rebuilt and reinforced until
it could truly break the awesome force
of the sea. Today, mooring space in the
harbour of Vestmannaeyjar is about one
mile.

The islanders were among the first to
import a rescue craft to the country.
They founded the Vestmannaeyjar Rescue Society in 1918, and it purchased a
steamship, which arrived in 1920. It was
considered a great financial accomplish-
ment at the time. This ship, besides ass-
isting boats in distress, was also used to
guard the territorial waters — not an
unnecessary task in those years, when

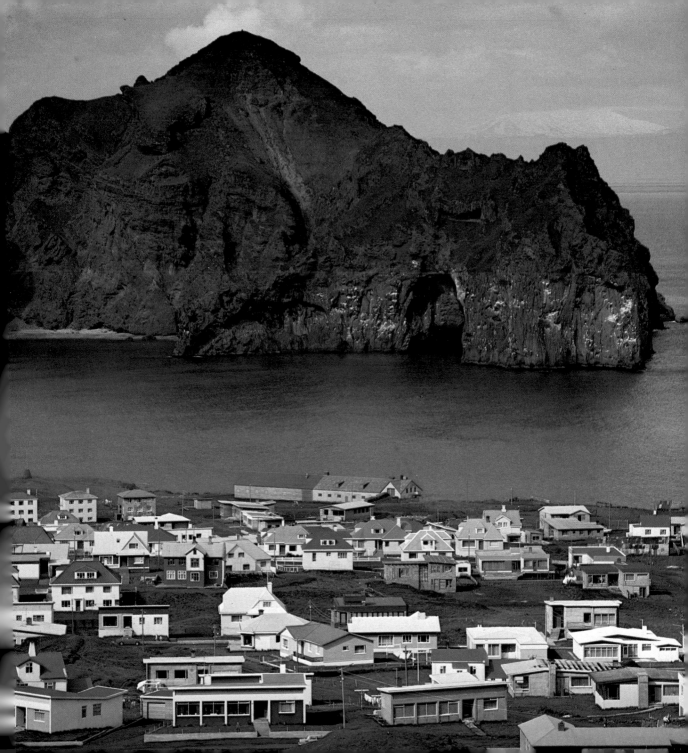

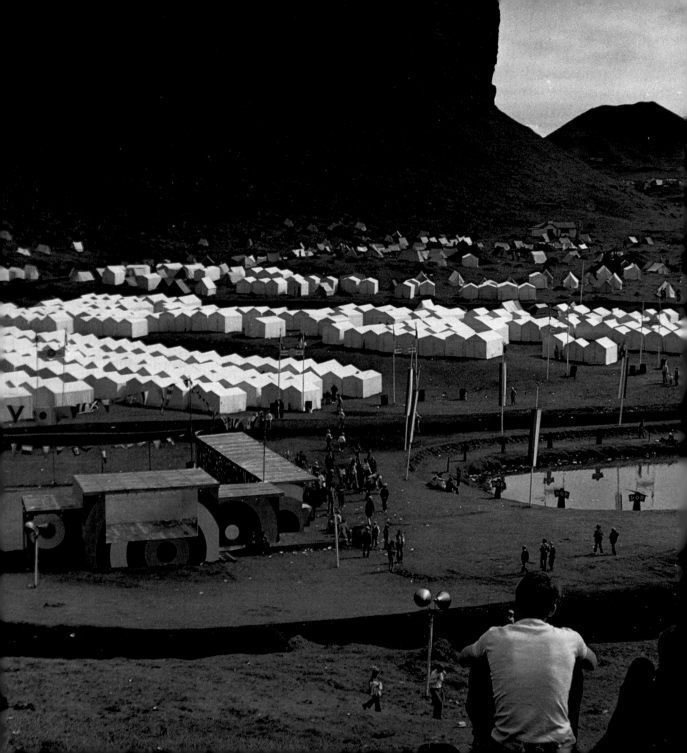

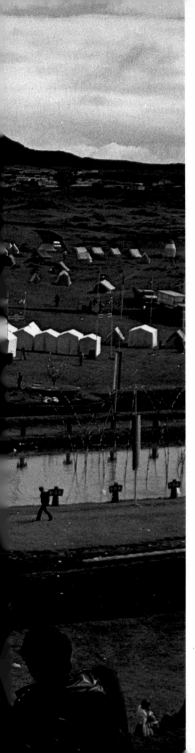

The National Festival in Vestmannaeyjar in the middle of summer attracts people from many parts. Then most of the inhabitants move to a beautiful valley outside town and stay there a couple of days in mirth and jollity. Everybody lives in a tent.

foreign fishing vessels in Icelandic waters were so aggressive that the local boats had no peace to lay their nets. What is more, the foreign vessels would trawl right up to the shoreline, killing young fish in such numbers that the best fishing grounds of the Icelandic boats were threatened with depletion. In 1926, the state took over the outfitting of this ship; it was the beginning of the Icelandic Coast Guard.

A long list of such examples could be compiled, attesting to the vigour and initiative of this small community. After the telephone had been introduced to Iceland in 1906, the islanders also sought to enjoy its convenience, but the state treasury pleaded poverty. Then, as before, the islanders took matters into their own hands. They founded a Telephone and Telegraph Company in 1911, laid a submarine cable out to Heimaey, as well as local lines, and thereby gained direct communication with the mainland network. Today, telephone service in the islands is among the best in the country. No fresh water is to be found in Vestmannaeyjar, much less waterfalls that could be harnessed to produce electricity. But the islanders established their own electric company, which began operations in 1916. The power was produced by a diesel plant, with an original generating capacity of 50 kilowatts; the present capacity is 5,700 kilowatts. It was not until 1962 that a submarine electric cable from the mainland was laid out to the islands. Still, sufficient emergency power was needed because of the constant

danger that the cable might break. The old plant, therefore, was kept operational. From the very first, the lack of water has been the great problem of the islanders. All the fish passing through the processing plants used to be cleaned with chlorinated sea water, while for personal consumption there was little else than rainwater gathered from the roofs. But it does not rain all the time, so the lack of domestic water was often keenly felt. In 1966, therefore, the islanders had an aqueduct built from a mountain reservoir on the mainland, some 14 miles from the coast, and from there a submarine double pipeline was laid the 8.5 miles out to the islands. The project was completed at a cost of more than $400 for every man, woman, and child in the community.

Transportation to and from the islands used to be quite difficult. Shipping was, originally, the only means, but sometimes the islands were isolated for days, or even weeks, because of violent weather. Now, there is a two-runway airport on Heimaey, where Icelandair's scheduled aircraft land every day, and the islanders have established their own airline.

Much has also been accomplished in terms of education and culture. The first formal elementary school in Iceland was established in Vestmannaeyjar in 1745. The islands now have a high school, a trade school, a nautical college, a music school, an art school, and an engineering school. There is a historical museum, a museum of natural history, and a good library. One of the country's most im-

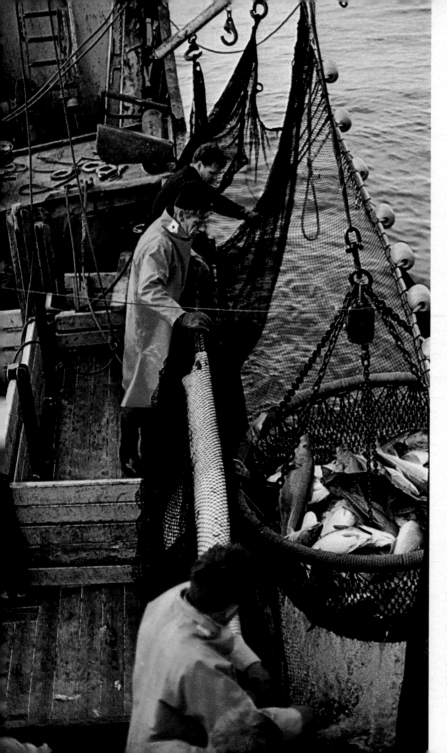

pressive modern hospitals is also located in Vestmannaeyjar, and there is a centre for preventive medicine.

It may be concluded, therefore, that the people of Vestmannaeyjar are an energetic lot. They have overcome difficult circumstances to create one of the most prosperous communities in Iceland. And the circumstances, in turn, have molded these people. Their manner is free and easy, as is often the case with those who by vigour and determination have made themselves independent and secured their livelihood, knowing no problem too big to surmount. Yet cooperation and helpfulness are deep-rooted in their nature. No one builds a house without the help of neighbours and friends. And in Vestmannaeyjar nearly everyone lives in a one-family house; there is olny a single apartment building. Another strong strand of their character is their belief in their land — the islands. Some mainlanders have thought that the islanders' sense of independence was close to local chauvinism. But those who have come to know them understand their desire to be dependent upon no one. They had to struggle for their living, and the struggle has been hard, albeit profitable. In recent years, the islanders have contributed more to the national product than any other comparable group of Icelanders. Prosperity in Vestmannaeyjar has also been greater than elsewhere in the country. There are more than 1,200 beautiful homes, with furnishings and modern appliances such as few in Iceland can boast, and more than 800 automobiles.

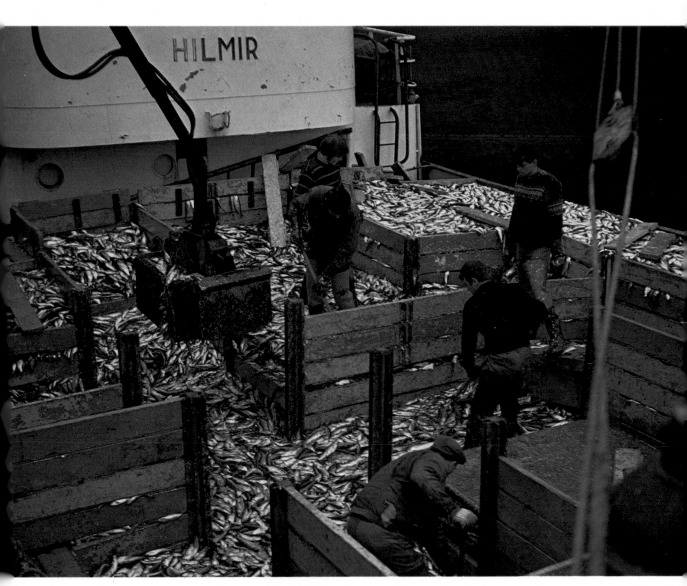

23

The people of Vestmannaeyjar constitute only about 2.5 percent of the Icelandic nation, but in recent years they have produced on the average about 11 percent, by value, of the country's exports — five times more per person than the average in other parts of the country. In 1960, the islanders produced a record 16 percent of the total exports, so the value of this community for the nation as a whole is by no means small.

One aspect of life in Vestmannaeyjar must not be forgotten, and that is the so-called national festival, which has been celebrated almost every year since 1874. It is held in a beautiful valley named Herjólfsdalur, where the first settler of the islands, Herjólfur, is said to have lived. The valley is actually an old volcanic crater. During the earliest festivals there would be a communal dinner al fresco. For that purpose an immense table was built out of rocks and turf, at which everybody sat together to partake of the meal. Now, most of the population virtually moves out to Herjólfsdalur, putting up tents for the three days of the festival, held in August. Hundreds of visitors also attend this celebration. Here they gather, side by side, labourers and board directors, truckdrivers and bankers, to sing, play, dance and simply have fun. The valley is beautifully decorated to resemble the setting of a fairy-tale. So, in the old crater, the struggle against the stormy seas in forgotten for a while, and that is how it has been for nearly one hundred years.

A Year of Thirteen Moons

People in Vestmannaeyjar greeted New Year, 1973, in the traditional manner. Families gathered in their homes at supper time for pork roasts or legs of lamb; some ate puffin and sipping wine. The evening passed in conversation and entertainment, and at midnight, when the church bells chimed farewell to the old year, welcoming the new one, and the steam whistles of the ships hooted along, the islanders sang the Icelandic equivalent of „Auld Lang Syne," kissed, and wished each other happiness in the new year, giving thanks for whatever good the old one had brought.

A good fishing season was expected. Enormous shoals of capelin were known to be migrating up to the Icelandic coast, and many boat-owners were preparing their vessels for trawling and seining. Faulty equipment was repaired; the boats were scraped and painted. Fish-meal factories and freezing plants, some of the most advanced in the country, were ready for work at full capacity. There was no reason to worry about the future; life in the islands demanded a great deal of work, but it also yielded ample rewards. Young married couples estimated their incomes for the year, reviewed building plans for their new houses, and made arrangements for the births of their children. Some even resolved to stop smoking or to abstain from liquor. The first half of January passed just like any other time of the year, and all was well. Old men, however, pointed out that 1973 was a year of 13 moons; it would see

When the boats are in, there is bustling activity around the harbour. The womenfolk stroll there with their baby carriages in order to meet their husbands who frequently have very short stop ashore. Who does not know the stories of 'the big one' that got away

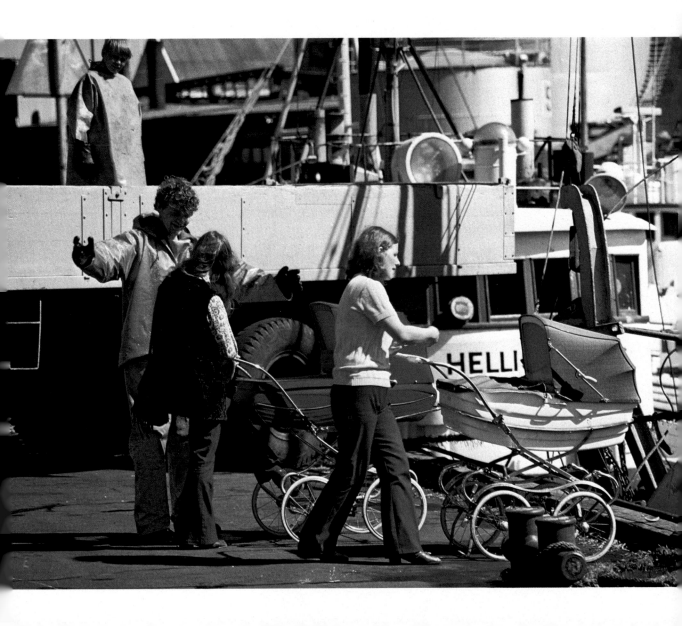

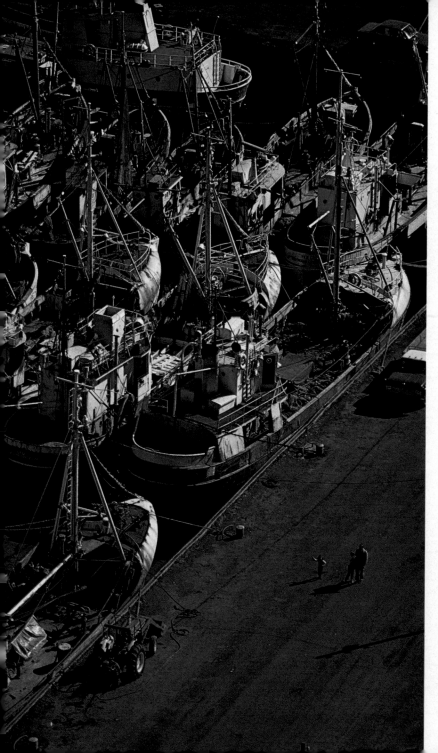

When the fishermen stay ashore, the boats are tied to the piers and the time used for mending and renewing the equipment. It was necessary to have everything in good shape in stormy weather, for the entrance to the harbour could be very difficult indeed (right).

full moons 13 times, including twice in June, on the first and the last day. This, they said, had always been considered a bad omen; in a year of 13 moons events of great magnitude would occur. But who listens to the chatter of old men in times of moon-walks and other technical miracles? Even though predictions and dream revelations generally tickle the mystic nerve of the Icelander, people tend to ignore such portents.

Everything appeared normal. The weather had been unusually good, and a fishing season of great promise was ahead. There was much talk about the extension to 50 nautical miles of the Icelandic fisheries limit, and the people of Vestmannaeyjar, just like other Icelanders, hoped that the resultant protection of the fish stocks would eventually increase them and thereby secure future catches. Then came January 22. As usual, the people of Vestmannaeyjar woke up early that Monday, perhaps with the exception of some who had been celebrating the night before. The winter morning was still dark as people walked to their work along the quiet streets. Children grabbed their breakfast and books and were off to school. Housewives began their chores, some of them dropping in on neighbours for a cup of coffee and a bit of gossip before they began preparing lunch. As it dawned, the boats could be seen in the harbour, where most of them lay moored. The weather was bad this morning, and the fleet had not gone out. Many visiting boats had also sought lee in port; the sea around the islands was

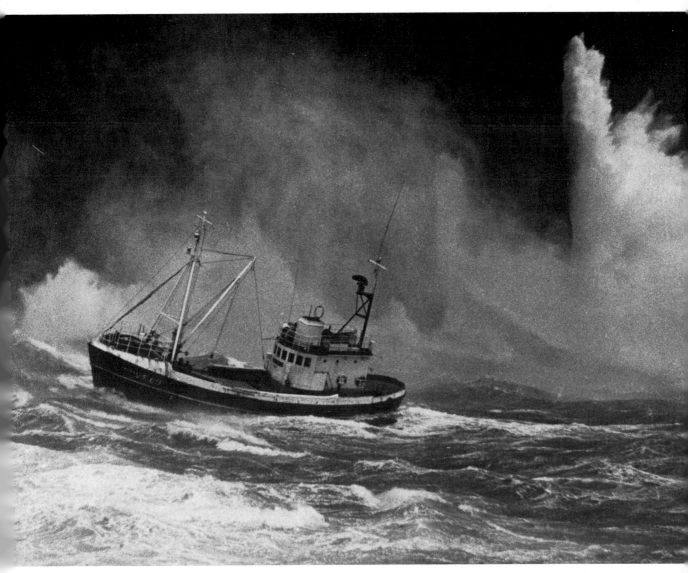

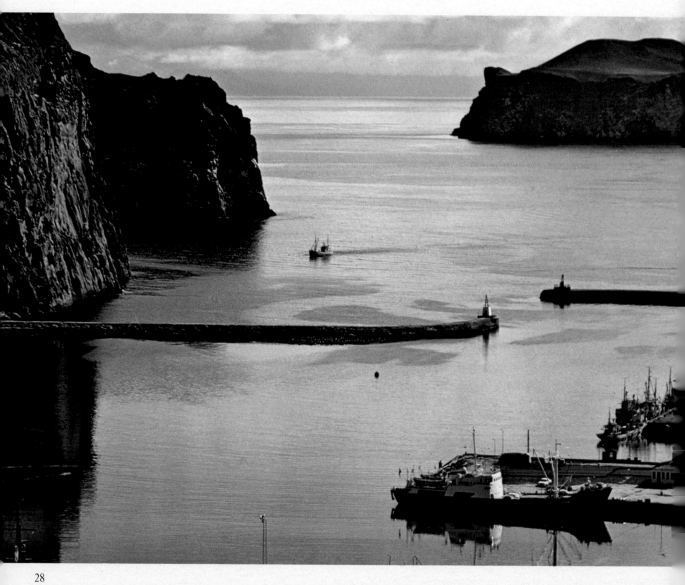

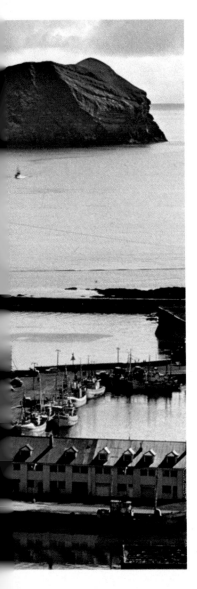

foaming white. Shortly before 2:00 p. m. a bulletin reported that a boat had been hit by heavy seas and badly damaged. In Vestmannaeyjar, the wind velocity reached 75 miles per hour, but such weather is no surprise to the islanders, and the day passed as usual. Toward evening, the wind began to taper off, and after supper, by the time people were sitting in their living rooms, watching television or talking about the day's events, the weather had become relatively quiet. Down at the harbour, the screaming birds could again be heard above the soughing of the wind; by midnight, total calm had come. Some people thought they felt an earth tremour or two during the evening, but that again was no more unusual than the gale.

After midnight, nocturnal peace enveloped the town, and few persons were out of doors. Gradually, the lights in the windows went out; tomorrow was another workday, and people needed sleep. In one house a birthday party was still going on, and merry laughter and song carried out to the street. Several men were on duty at the police station, the telephone office, and the navigational radio station, and the guards at the processing plants were making their rounds of inspection to see that everything was in order. The time was approaching 2:00 a.m. Two men went for a good-weather stroll to the eastern part of town, enjoying the sound of the sea rippling gently at the shore after the roaring surf of the day. Someone was also driving up by Helgafell, the old volcanic cone, which

had lain dormant for 5,000 or 6,000 years.

It was now close to 2:00 a.m. The town was tranquil, but just to the east of it the ground began to quiver slightly. Pebbles were thrown up in the air, as if they had been lying on a taut skin which someone had struck lightly. Then the surface of the land appeared to swell up, and soon it began to crack. It was as if a sharp knife were being drawn over the flesh of the earth and blood were beginning to spurt. Only, it was not blood; it was fire and embers. In a matter of minutes, nearly a mile-long fissure opened, running from north-northeast to south-southwest. Lava immediately began to well out of it, and glowing cinders squirted high into the air. The fissure consisted of dozens of eye-like small craters, forming a continuous row of fire east of the town. At the north-northeastern end of it, which reached all the way down to the sea, the fire was very close to the easternmost houses. From there, the crack ran south-southwestward on the east side of Helgafell, directly across the eastern part of the island, reaching the sea at that end also. Witnesses do not agree exactly when the eruption began, but most maintain it was at 1:55 a.m. The clock on Town Hall stopped at that time, and it has not been going since.

And Suddenly One Night...

"There's Been an Eruption"

There were not many who witnessed the very beginning of the eruption; most people were already asleep. The two men strolling about the eastern section of town were probably the first to see the fire. They stopped short for a moment, gazing in astonishment at the sight they saw. For a few seconds they could not even think; they just stood there as if spellbound, staring at the grand spectacle. To all appearances, the fire was so close that it seemed likely to swallow the town in a short time. The idea struck them that Helgafell had exploded, and for a fraction of a second it also occurred to them that the eastern outskirts of the town had caught fire. When they finally realised what was happening, they ran home to wake their wives and children. In another part of town a man, looking out of his window, saw the sky lit up by flames; it did not take him long to understand that an eruption had begun. He awakened his wife and children, and they dressed in haste. He stuffed a good deal of money, which he had kept at home, in his pocket, and then hurried his family down to the harbour. Some people telephoned their relatives and friends in Reykjavík, telling them the news.

„There's been an eruption!"

„Don't you think it's a bit late for jokes?" retorted the man's brother in Reykjavík.

„But I'm not joking," said the islander. „There's an eruption just outside, and we're leaving the house."

„OK, so you've had one too many," re-plied the incredulous brother. It took the islander a long time to convince him, and many others had a similar reaction. Everybody was dumbfounded; people just could not believe their eyes or ears. Only a few seconds after the eruption started the phones began to ring in the police station and the fire department. People ran from house to house to in-form those who were still asleep of the situation. Then the fire signal was sound-ed, and police cars and fire trucks, sirens wailing, drove through town to rouse everybody. At first, those who had just fallen asleep did not know why they had been awakened. Some thought their house had caught fire or there had been a serious accident. But the rumble from the volcano soon told them the truth. One man jumped out of bed and told his wife to dress their child, while he snatched a chunk of cheese and a leg of lamb from the refrigerator. With that safely tucked under his arm, he and his family left their house.

The eruption grew more violent during the first few minutes. As it reached a climax, the local authorities conferred in Town Hall to decide what to do. They concluded at once that it would be safest to evacuate the island; no one knew what was to come. Orders were relayed all over town for everybody to gather down by the harbour.

Nearly all of the local boats, some sev-enty of them, were at the wharves; there were also many from other ports. The navigational radio station had transmit-ted the international distress call, „May-

This is how the fissure at the foot of Helgafell looked at dawn on January 23. The craters can be counted in the dozens, and they squirt fire and brimstone, as this aerial view clearly shows.

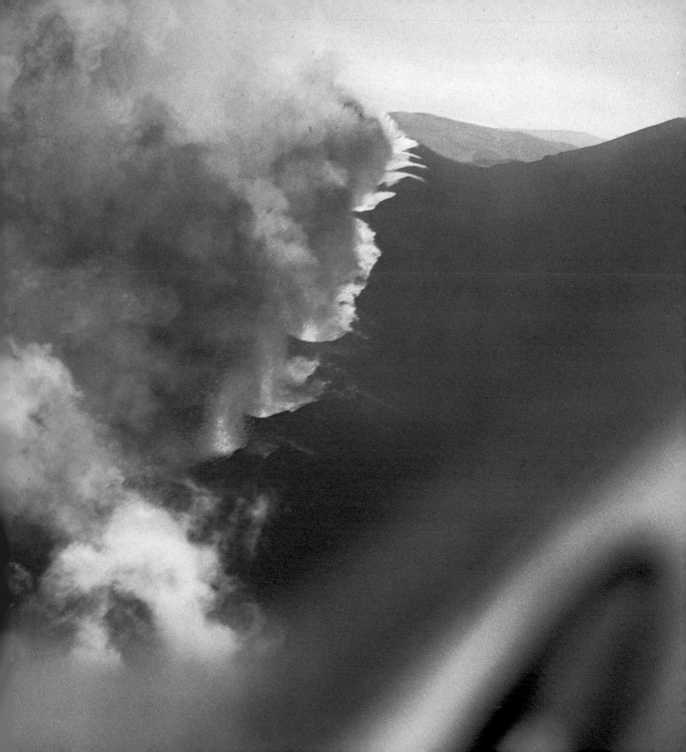

The rays of the sun try breaking through the pillar of ashes, creating an awesome impression. Silhouetted against the sky is Helgafell, silently observing the fury (below). On the opposite page, a dense cloud of steam is seen rising thousands of feet towards the sky. This was only the beginning.

On the following pages, a picture taken from Helgafell of the fissure on the morning of that fateful day. Here can be seen more clearly than in most pictures the proximity of the volcanic activity to the edge of the town, which was soon to be burned down and shattered by the lava.

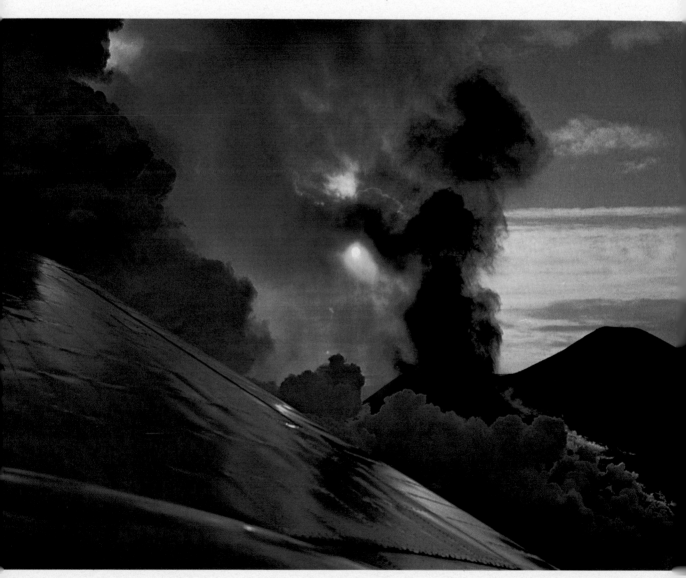

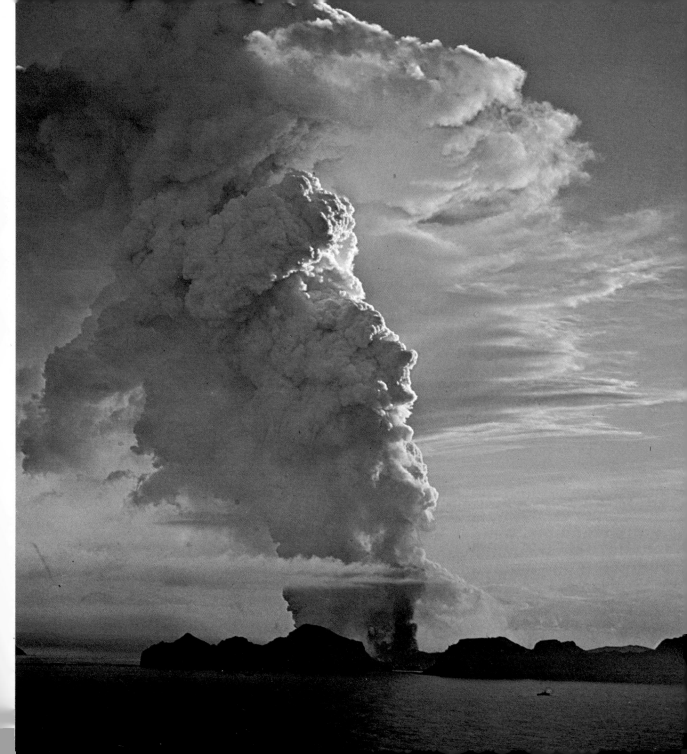

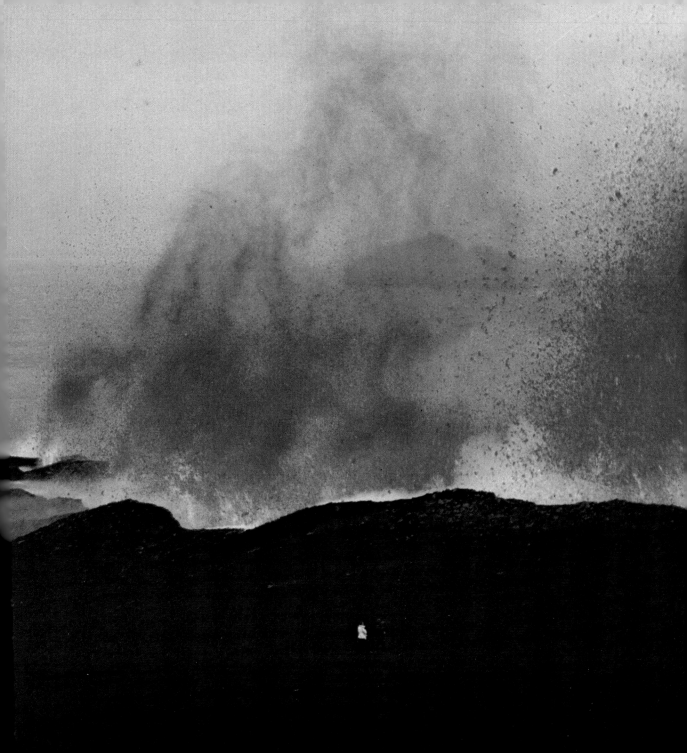

day," announcing the eruption. Boats fishing in the vicinity of the islands immediately hauled in their gear and set course for Heimaey. More and more people were emerging from their homes. The news had gone through town with incredible speed, and everybody seemed to be taking it with amazing composure. Most people tried to take along a few necessities, such as bedding and clothing. The children were bundled up in warm clothes, and then people left for the unknown. The crowd in the streets grew steadily, everybody headed toward the harbour. Many used their cars to get there, leaving them on the piers. The men helped women, children, and old people aboard, and as soon as the boats were loaded, they cast off for the mainland.

The government in Reykjavík had been consulted in order to organise the rescue operation, but actually the people themselves presided over their evacuation, for they did only what seemed natural under the circumstances. The first boat left the harbour only minutes after the eruption began; no one was heard demanding to be on it. Then the departures continued, one after another, and those standing on the quays became fewer and fewer. Every attempt was made to make people comfortable aboard the boats, for the voyage would take about four hours. Most people had tried to leave their houses in order — to put out lights, turn off burners, and lock up. A few forgot. Some preparations had to be made for those who were not ambulatory — the

sick and the old. As many as possible were dressed in warm, windproof clothes, but they had to wait for planes.

In Reykjavík the wheels began turning. The first plane was in the island about an hour after the eruption began. Traffic control personnel were ready in the little tower at the airport. At first it was feared that the main runway was out of service; some large pieces of pumice had fallen at the eastern end of it, which was not far from the fissure. Fortunately, this fear proved unfounded, and the air was soon resounding with the noise of aircraft. Large passenger carriers from Icelandair landed, taking off with the sick and the old. Helicopters and cargo planes from the U.S. Defense Force at Keflavík Airport participated in the rescue operation. Everything went quickly and smoothly; within hours the hospital was empty.

Those who first arrived at the Vestmannaeyjar by planes that night will never forget the sight that met their eyes. Midway between the mainland and the islands they could see the pillars of fire rising from the fissure. They counted more than forty. From the distance it looked like some of the lava was spouting out of Helgafell, but it proved to be from the crack east of the mountain. Helgafell was silhouetted against the wall of fire like a black cone, and below the blazing inferno cowered the town. It all seemed so unreal and incredible. There were lights in windows, and the street lamps flickered. Down by the harbour, considerable commotion could be seen,

The houses in the easternmost part of the town stand close to the heaps of pumice which were formed during the first hour of the eruption. This is an incredible sight but was to become familiar.

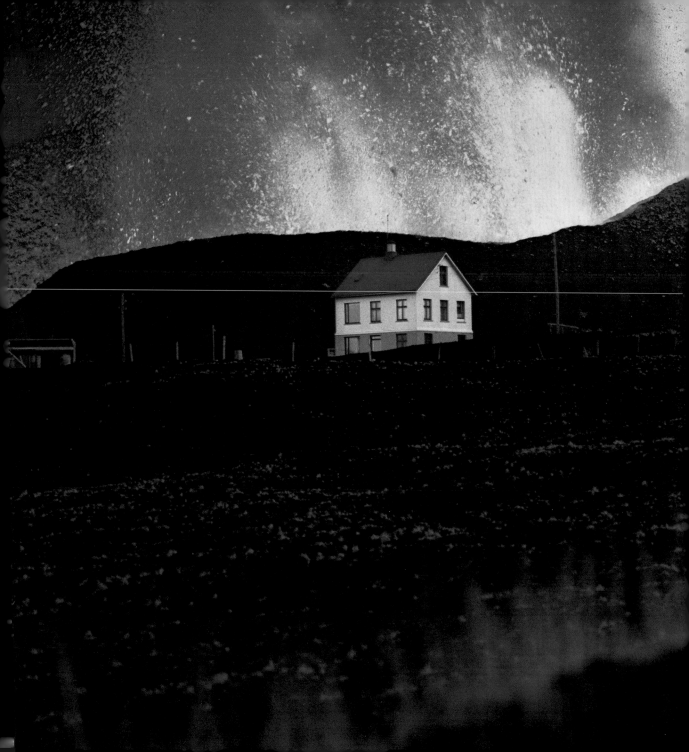

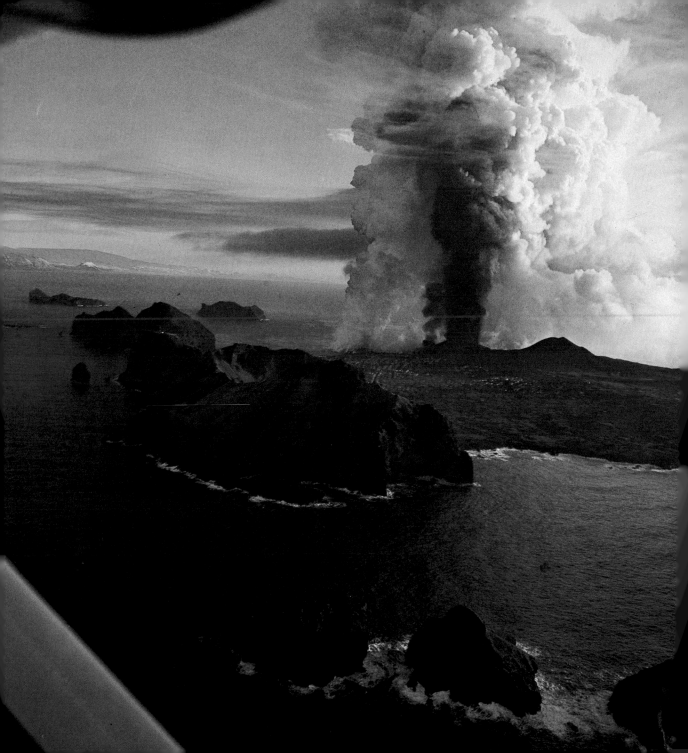

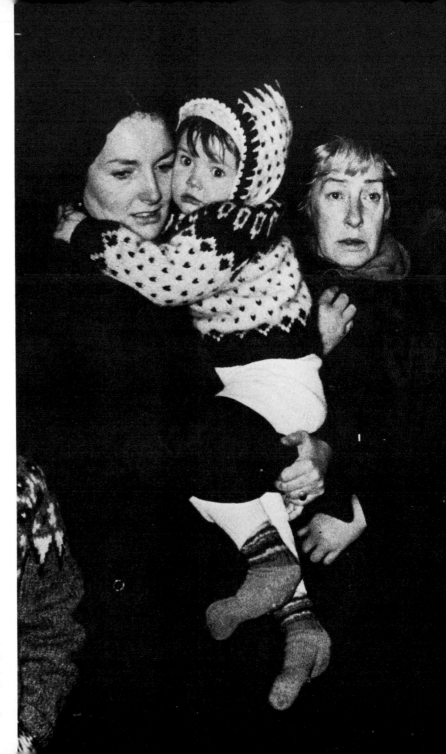

and out at sea the lights of the numerous boats, headed for the mainland, were visible; they resembled a floating city.

The airport was bustling and busy; planes were coming and going without cessation. Almost every airworthy craft in Reykjavík went to the islands that night and the following day. Everybody wanted to contribute to the rescue operation, and no questions were asked about the length of the working day or remuneration. The entire nation took part in the events happening in the Vestmannaeyjar. From the earliest times, Icelanders have had to face the fact that theirs is a volcanic country and eruptions do not preannounce their arrival. They have caused unmeasured miseries — loss of life and property, the devastation of flourishing districts, where green fields have been turned into desolate wastelands. Such events have impressed upon a small nation, which has had to fight hard for its existence, the necessity of standing together as one. There have been times when the very life of the Icelanders in their own country hung in the balance. But they have continued living, and it is their faith in the country which has given them the courage to go on. Now, once again their solidarity was being tested.

An Atmosphere of Eeriness

During the first hours of the eruption everything happened so quickly that it is hard to make out single events. What was most miraculous was that only five or six hours after the initial outburst, most of the islanders were safely on the

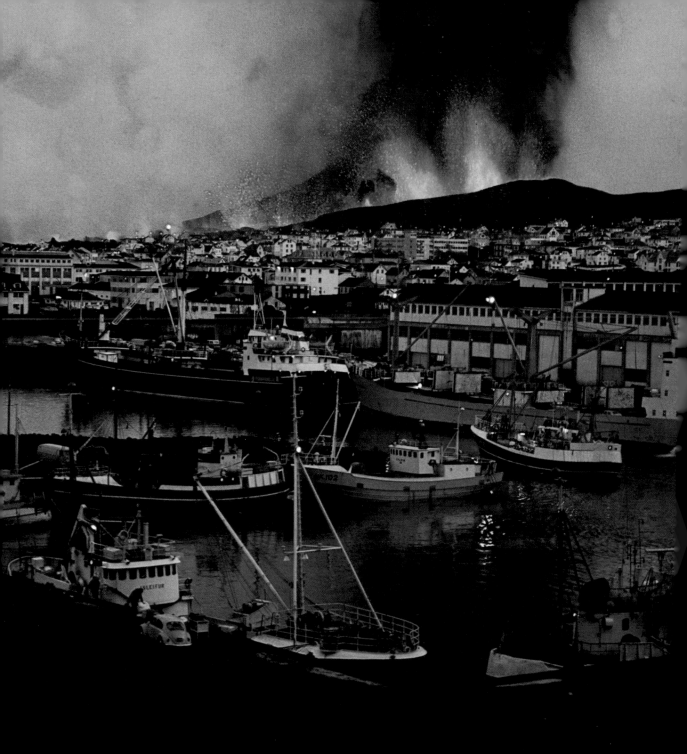

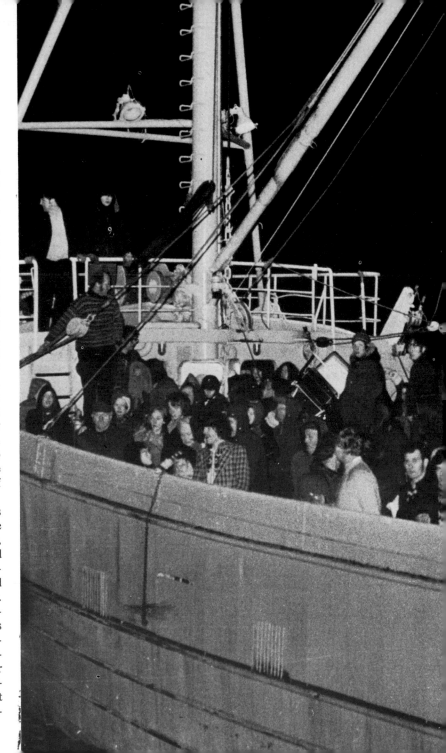

The evacuation is in full swing. Ships and boats transport people and goods to the mainland, to safer shores.

mainland. The evacuation went like a well-greased machine, even though no previous plan existed for what to do in a natural calamity of this sort. The smoothness of the operation is attributable, primarily, to the calm, unruffled manner of the inhabitants. Those who know say that the proximity for three years to the eruption of Surtsey had much to do with how sensibly people responded. They had seen how eruptions behaved, and the closeness to one had become as natural as an everyday affair. An incredible number of islanders did not want to leave that first night. And when the removal of furnishings began, it was good to have vigorous men who knew the place already. Some elderly men did not want to leave at all, saying they had lived on the island all their lives, and if it was to perish, they wanted to go with it. No one was forced to leave Heimaey — only asked for the sake of safety.

When newsmen arrived, some two hours after the eruption began, a considerable number of people were at the airport, waiting for passage. Ambulances and police cars, their emergency lights spinning, were busily transporting sick and old people from the town to the airport. Planes were waiting on the runway, propellers turning, and took off as soon as they were filled to capacity. An old woman, born in Vestmannaeyjar, was leaving her island for the first time in her life. No doubt she must have asked herself whether she would ever return. But she said nothing, just thanked her ·rescu-

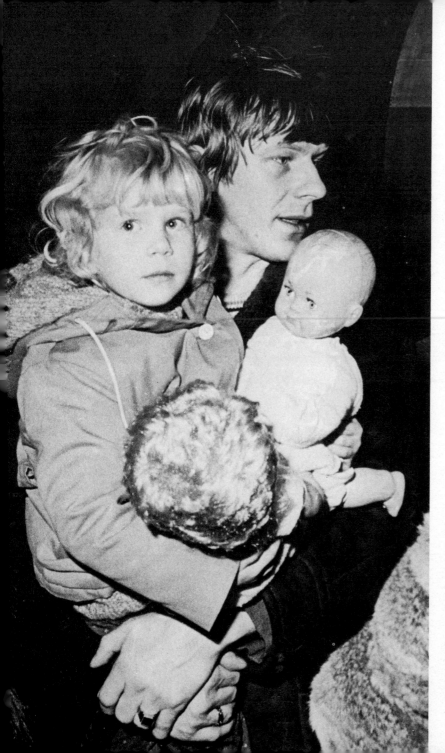

ers for the lift and boarded the plane. The young men taking their wives and children over to the mainland were already wondering when they would be able to return; no failing hearts there. What had happened, no one could control; it had to be endured.

Driving into town in the darkness, one could see a red sheen flickering on the gables and walls of the houses, and the rumble from the eruption echoed from the cliffs around the harbour. Only a few people were visible in the streets, most of them seeing to their property and preparing for the salvage of their household articles. The force of the eruption was enormous, and from time to time the town shuddered as if trying to shake off this unwelcome visitation. The pumice was carried out to sea by a northwesterly wind, but some had fallen over the eastern periphery of the town.

In Town Hall the council was still in session, trying to decide a course of action. Should everybody, without exception, be sent to the mainland for a few days, during which it might become clearer how the eruption would develop, or would it be wiser to begin immediately vacating both residential and industrial buildings, which meant maintaining a large corps of salvage workers on the island? Great responsibility rested on the shoulders of the councilmen. By keeping a salvage corps, they might be literally risking the lives of hundreds of people. By evacuating everybody they would be signing the surrender, and that was not consistent with their temperament. Those

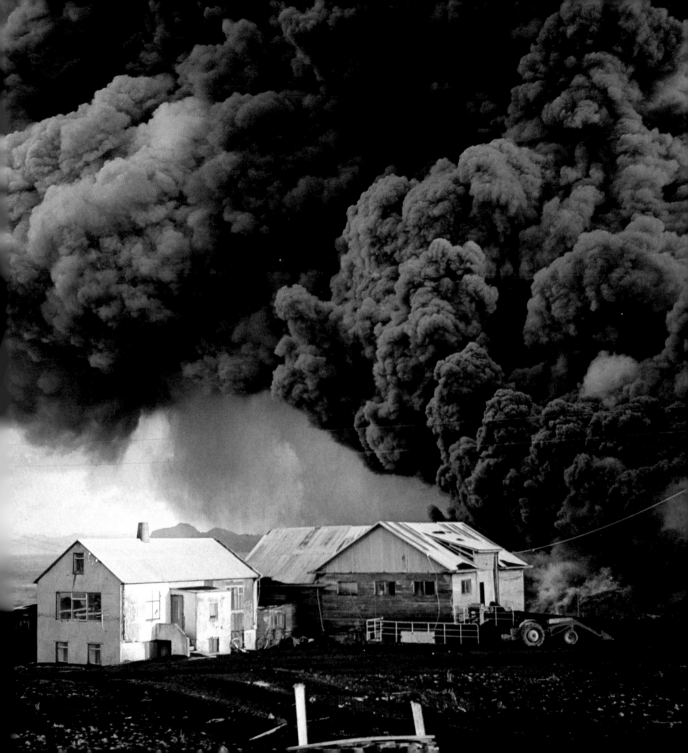

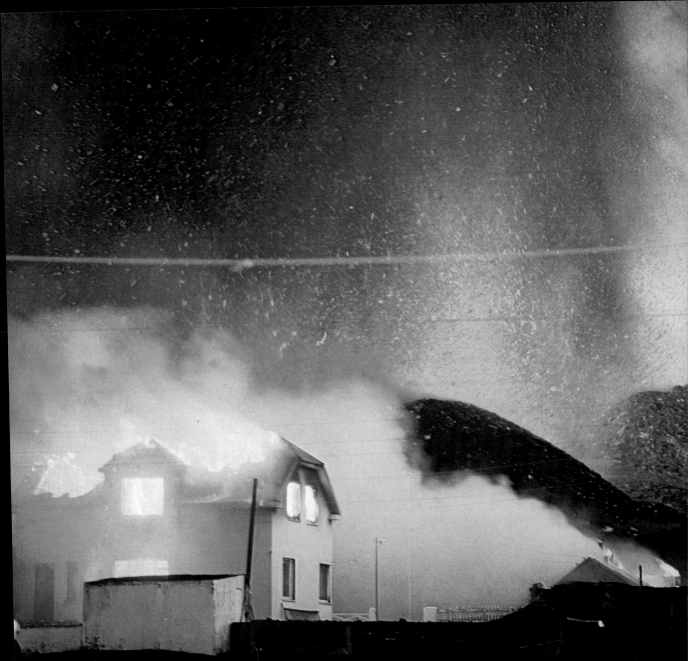

A flaming splatter of lava has penetrated the roof of a house and instantly ignited it. The sick and the old were moved away in helicopters the very first night. The picture on the following pages is a nocturnal one and gives a peculiar impression of the helplessnes of the people and the insufficiency of human endeavours in the face natural catastrophes.

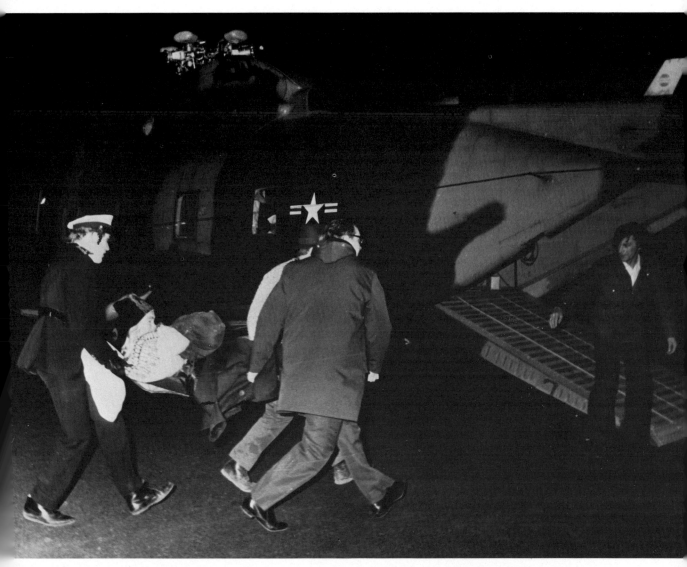

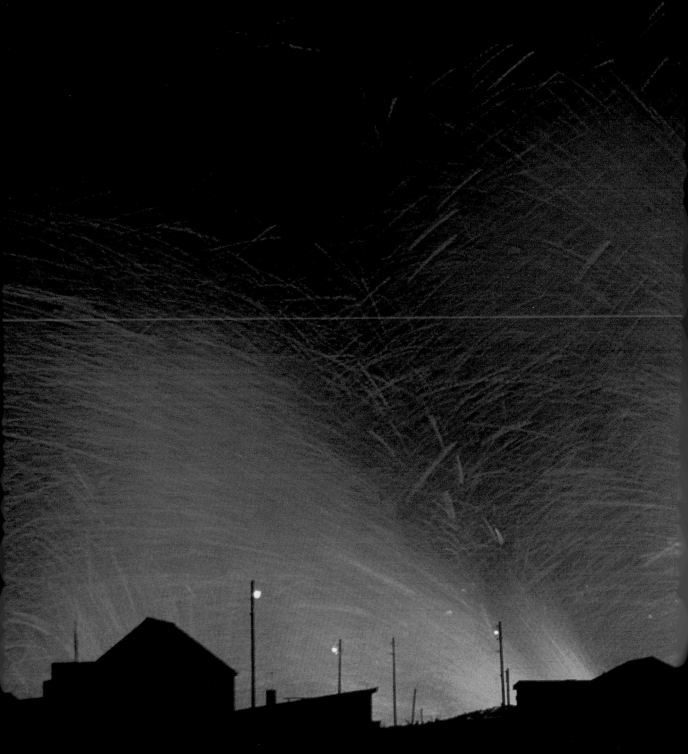

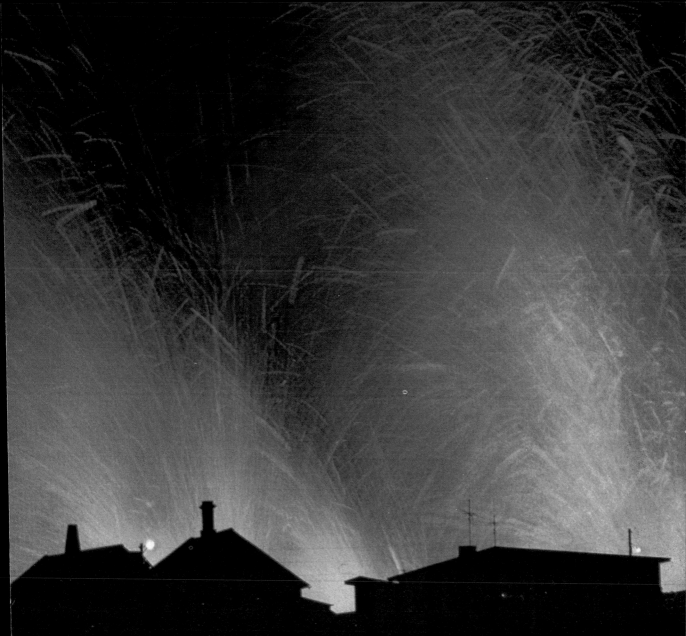

who wanted to stay were allowed to. There seemed to be no great hazard for the time being; the direction of the wind was favourable, property was not in immediate danger, and somehow it evolved that each decided for himself to persevere.

Walking about the streets of the town that first night, one was reminded of stories of ghost ships, found drifting at sea, with no explanation why the crew had abandoned them. Here, however, the explanation lay on everybody's doorstep. In some of the deserted houses, there were lights in every window, and even the front doors were open. Many had forgotten their pets, or they had been outside when the eruption began. Here and there a cat was meowing at the door of a house now empty of people, while dogs ran to whomever they saw moving about. Some people had let out their sheep and horses before they left. The animals stood there motionless, staring at the fire. One horse went mad with fright and ran toward the fire. He had the hair singed off his hide, but not too seriously, and he survived. Even the birds were affected. At first they flew off, farther into the island, and their screeching was silenced. But once they became accustomed to the rumbling noise, they turned back and hovered over the harbour, looking for food. Everything was pervaded by a feeling of mystery, an atmosphere of eeriness no one can understand, except those who were there.

More like Fiction than Truth

The ministers of the Icelandic government were awakened and told the news shortly after the eruption began. The State Civic Defense Committee was immediately summoned to a meeting at its headquarters, an underground bunker in Reykjavik's principal police station. There, sheltered by thick steel walls, which are supposed to provide protection against consequences of a nuclear explosion, the committee members gathered around a large table. It took them some time to realise fully the magnitude of the problem, but once they had, they acted swiftly. Icelandic Red Cross personnel were also at work. First, it had to be decided how to transport more than 4,000 persons from the port of Thorlákshöfn, where most of the Vestmannaeyjar boats berthed. It was resolved that all the city buses be appro- where they would be temporarily housed in the city's schools. Thorlákshöfn is about a 45-minute drive from Reykjavík, and the buses were there in time to pick up the people as they debarked. Some had become seasick on the way, but otherwise everybody was in good health. Infants were asleep in their parents' arms, unaware of what was happening. Little girls held their dolls or teddybears, and some of the boys had taken along their toy cars and boats. It was a silent crowd that boarded the buses, and many could not resist glancing back toward their islands, where the flickering glow from the fires could be discerned across the waters. The transportation from Thorlákshöfn took only a short time, and

The heap of pumice grows, and it is a though the eruption were taking place i the centre of town. Still, not everyone wa willing to leave his island

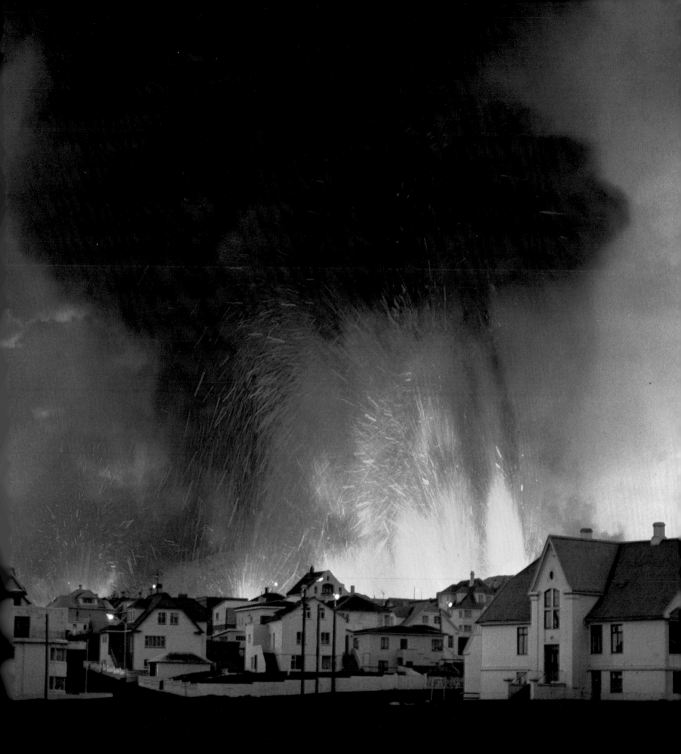

The pumice continues falling, and high-pressur
hoses have to be used in order to clear the wing
of the aircraft. Meanwhile, people try
precede the lava in getting the furnitu
(opposite

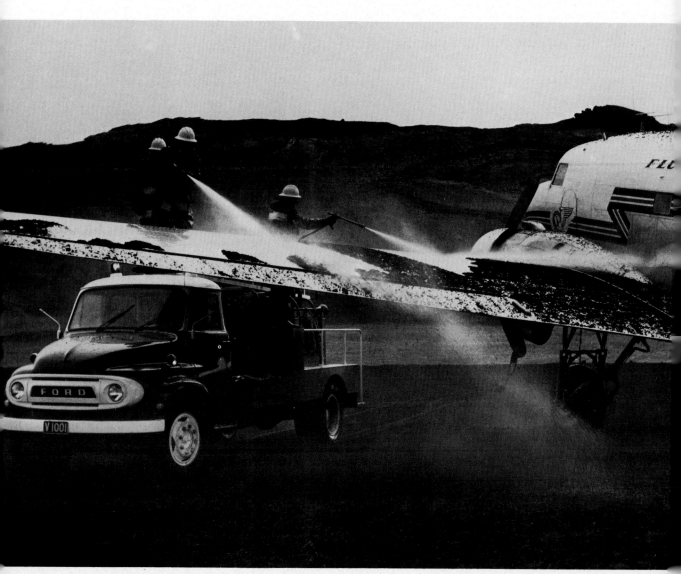

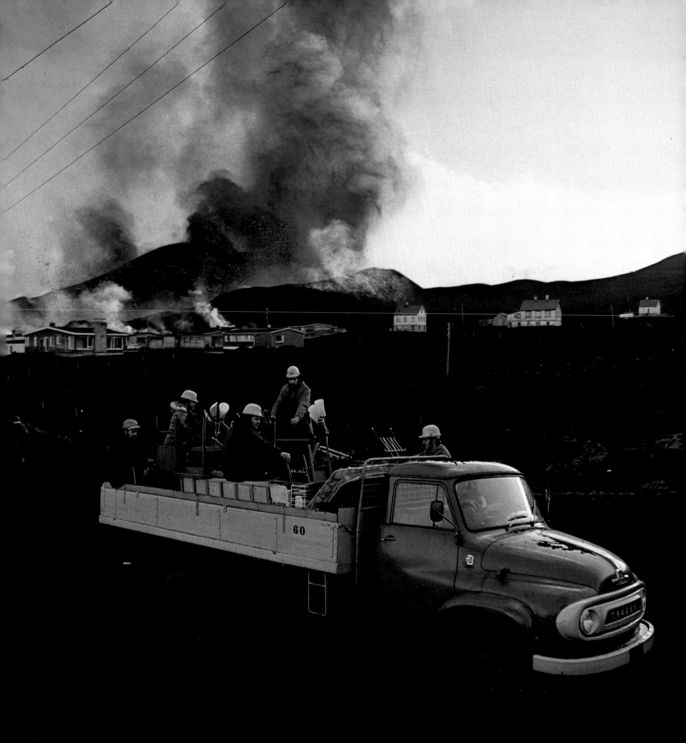

most of the people were put up in school buildings. Some large school and office cafeterias had already been opened, providing free food for the refugees. The State Broadcasting Service, which is usually on the air from 7:00 a.m. until midnight, was reopened with news from the islands immediately after the eruption became known. But there were few listeners; most people were sleeping. Many relatives of the islanders, however, had been awakened and were ready to receive their kinsfolk, when they arrived in the city toward morning. Icelanders in general did not know of the eruption before the scheduled news hour at 7:30 a. m. Nobody had expected anything unusual, so no one had turned on his radio before the regular time.

But once people knew, hundreds volunteered their assistance. And many were given jobs to do. The day of January 23 was not old when the bulk of those islanders, who had been housed in the schools, had secured lodgings in private homes. Such arrangements were not necessarily made with friends or relatives; many people, even those who did not have much space to spare, offered to take in anyone in need of it. That story will be long remembered in Iceland. Everybody understood the feelings of their countrymen, who had been forced to abandon everything they had — their beautiful homes, their work, their beloved islands — and now had nothing to look forward to but uncertainty. When people finally had time to think·about all that had happened, a whole community had

been transferred to a safe place; no life had been lost and no injury suffered. Little wonder that people felt it sounded more like fiction than truth.

A Life's Work Lost

When it began to dawn in Vestmannaeyjar on January 23, it was as if the eruption subsided. The fire looked less awesome when the darkness was no longer there to heighten its impact. Considerable changes soon took place at the site. The craters southwest of Helgafell ceased spewing, their force being combined in fewer vents northeast of the mountain, that is, directly above the eastern outskirts of the town. Here, the craters were constantly changing. As one opened with tremendous force, another vanished beneath the stream of lava. This continued all morning; sometimes four or five craters would be active, at other times only two or three. Large quantities of lava had been discharged overnight but had all run out to sea. A group of geologists, flown to the island during the night, were beginning their observations. The temperature of the lava was measured and proved to be more than 1000 centigrades. The lava was not too thin but crept onward slowly and continuously; the island had already been considerably enlarged. Much volcanic material had piled up in a ridge, and where formerly there had been clear view out to sea, the line of sight was now blocked by pumice and lava. Changes in the eruption site were so rapid that it was difficult to identify any landmarks.

The ruins of burnt-down houses increas
in number, and the lava advances. Th
fire from the craters reddens the hal
ruined house-gable

52

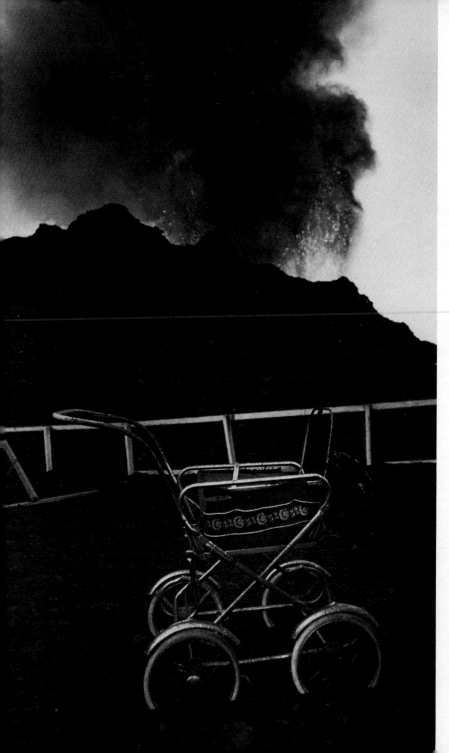

As the day wore on, a large forceful vent suddenly opened up just above the few easternmost houses, and lava from it began to move in the direction of the town. Though not swift-flowing, its forward edge was soon uncomfortably close to the nearest houses. In one of these lived a old farmer, who had spent his strength during a long, active life cultivating fields of grass, so that he might run a farm with sheep and cattle. Here he had pulled the rocks from the ground with his callused hands and carted them off in order to enlarge his fields. His relatives lived in six other houses in the neighbourhood. This old man could do nothing when his fields were covered with pumice and the lava flow began to threaten his house. For a brief moment he gave vent to his emotions, then acknowledged the fact: no one would farm there any more. He let his cows out of the barn and drove them to a place near the harbour, where all of them were slaughtered. The elements had won the first round, but the old man was still determined to return.

That morning boats continued going back and forth between the islands and the mainland. Many skippers, remembering there was an important fishing season ahead, began to remove their nets and other equipment. A few boats, lacking their engines, were in the harbour at the time; they were towed away. A number of fishermen also began to transport their possessions, and such activities increased as the day passed. Large cargo ships were sent to the islands in order to

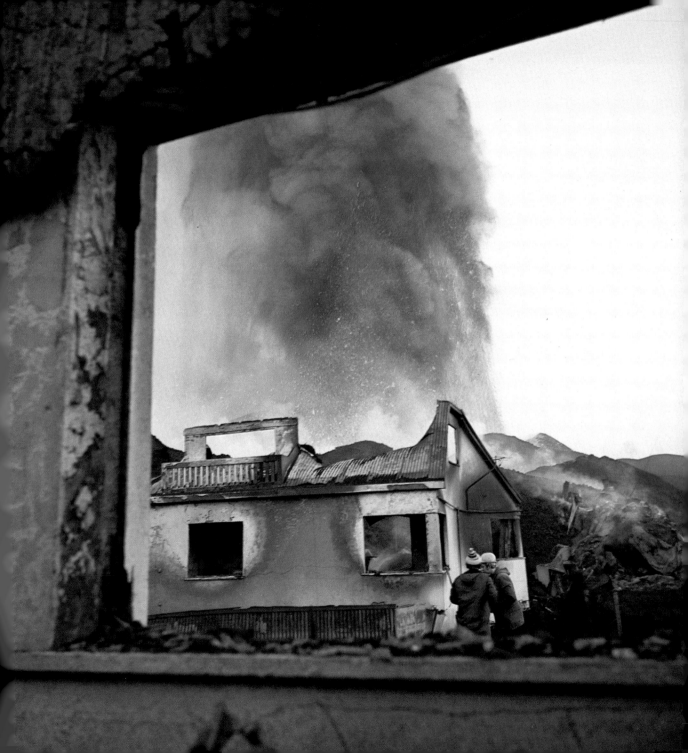

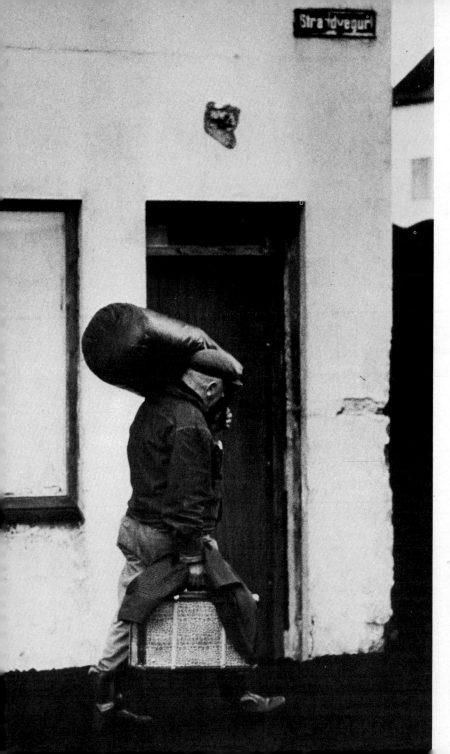

Straudvegur

Most people carried what they could, but heavier things had also to be removed from these houses, among them modern appliances like freezers, refrigerators, and washing machines (opposite), which wait at the pier for transportation to the mainland.

take automobiles to the mainland. From the easternmost houses, which were in imminent danger, furniture and appliances were also salvaged. In this part of town were many extraordinarily handsome new one-family homes which young people, with the help of their neighbours, had used every spare hour to erect. These were now emptied as far as possible, and their contents taken by trucks down to the harbour, where they were either put aboard boats or into storage. It was very difficult for many of these homeowners to accept the fact that they would have to abandon their houses perhaps for good. They carried out their belongings without packing them: refrigerators, freezers, washing machines, and television sets were loaded on the trucks. Clothes were put into plastic bags or boxes, and the kitchen cupboards were swept clean. While one of the houses was being thus evacuated, burning spatters of lava began to fall all around it, posing considerable danger to the salvage people. Some did not bother about carpets or shelving systems, perhaps hoping that they would be able to return. One after another, the trucks made their way to the harbour, loaded with furniture; many pepole did not even have the time to label their articles. During these transports personal property suffered heavy damage. Some owners said that by the time their belongings reached the mainland, up to half of them had been ruined. In some cases, the furniture was first moved to warehouses located at the harbour and then aboard the boats, which sometimes

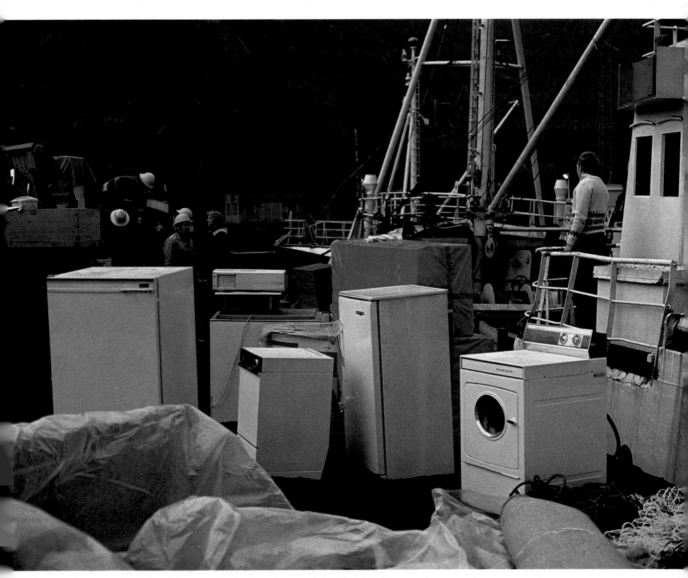

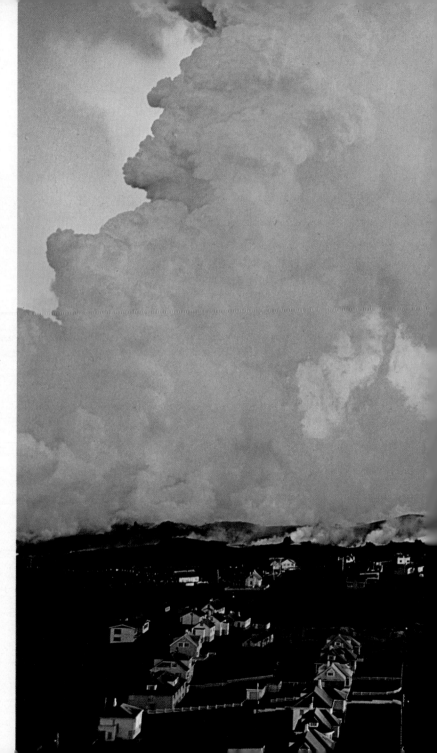

were battered by seas on the way over to the mainland. There, the furniture was again put into storage until the owner had secured a permanent dwelling. It is easy to imagine how white enameled refrigerators and delicate furniture must have looked after such travels. But people continued to move; to begin with it was their main occupation.

That day the first house on Heimaey burned to the ground. It was only the beginning; there was more to come. The house was ignited when a flaming splatter of lava landed on the roof, blazed a hole through it, and fell into the living room. The fire caught on in no time, and the house turned into a blistering furnace. Only minutes before, the last chair had been carried out of it. When this happened, the most violent crater was just above the house. The volcanic crack had lengthened northeastward out to sea, and two heaps of pumice were rising out of the waters. There was bubbling and seething all around, and a great column of vapour sizzled toward the sky. It had begun to drizzle, and the smoke and the vapour blended with the low-hanging rain clouds in a cover of darkness.

Some 300 men were on the island that day, and everything was ready for emergency departure in case the situation worsened. Spatters of lava, bursting almost ceaselessly into the air, fell all around the crater and onto the nearest houses. The speed of the lava current was similar to that of a quiet-flowing river, and the stream carried with it rocks and

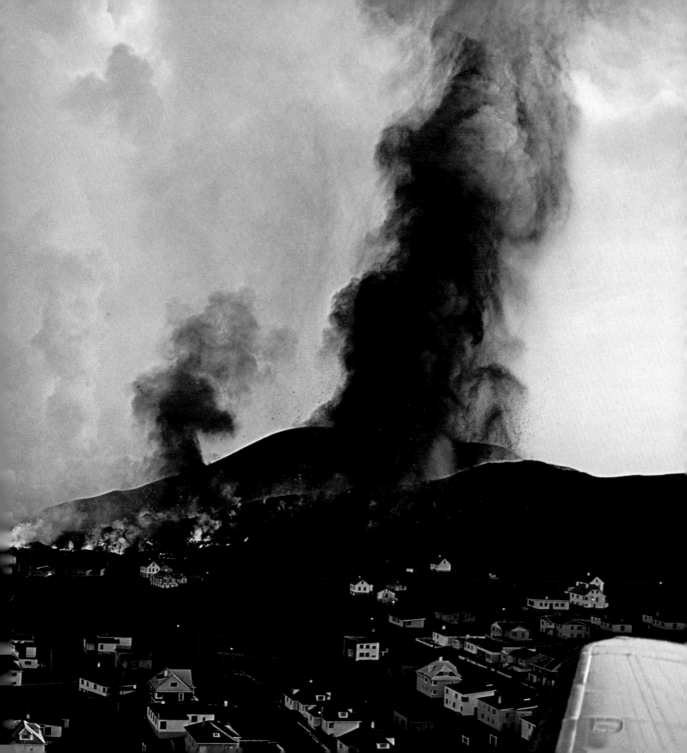

boulders measuring some 25—30 feet in diameter.

So passed this day. There was no appreciable change in the force of the eruption. It was as if all this awesome power was trying to find itself a definite channel instead of popping up here and there as it had done so far. People continued to move their belongings, and ships arrived to transport products from the freezing plants — packaged and frozen seafood worth millions of dollars.

The Abomination of Destruction

The night before January 25 the principal authorities of Vestmannaeyjar held a meeting at which it was decided, with the consent of the State Civic Defense Committee, that the islanders themselves should have the power to determine what to do about evacuating the people who had remained. In the evening, the direction of the wind had shifted to a southeasterly one, and large quantities of pumice were borne over most parts of the town. Several houses were soon ignited by the glowing cinders. The edge of the lava was also crawling closer, and the outlook was bad. More pumice fell. What happened during the night became clear in the morning. By that time, any movement about town was difficult because of the rain of volcanic materials, pieces of which were large enough to lacerate bare skin; nor was it entirely painless when they hit one's shoulders. The sight that met the eye at dawn can hardly be described in words. There was pumice and more pumice wherever one looked. A great deal had fallen in the centre of town; in the churchyard, the gravestones had nearly vanished, and the layer became gradually thicker as one approached the volcano. At one house an inventive owner had installed water hoses which continuously sprinkled the gable closest to the eruption. Here, the tops of the fence posts could barely be distinguished, and still farther on, the houses were practically disappearing under the heaps. There were places where the hills of pumice actually concealed whole houses, with telephone and electric lines vanishing into the mounds. Elsewhere, the ridge of a roof or the top part of a gable was still visible. Some electric lines, heated by the rain of cinders, had sagged under their own weight and were lying close to the surface. In this highest-lying section of town, two more houses had caught fire, the roof of one having caved in under the weight of the pumice; in the other, the fire was smouldering underneath the massive piles.

All morning long the pumice kept falling. During the most forceful spurts it was thrown so high into the air that it was cooled below freezing and fell down white with those previously fallen. The ruins of the houses that had burned the first day vanished under the lava that morning. Of two other houses that had burned nearby, the walls alone were left standing. A broken water pipe sent a jet of water gushing up in the air. In this neighbourhood also was a newly erected house in which every window pane had

The pumice spared no one, neither dead nor alive. This is what the cemetery looked like on the morning of 27 January, only four days after the eruption started. Later, it entirely disappeared.

60

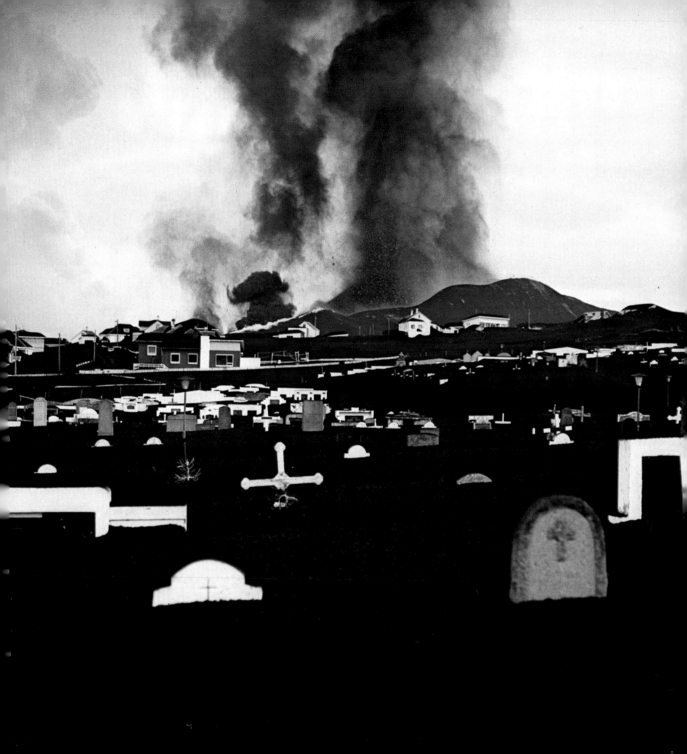

The houses were gradually submerged, but the rescue work was continued and the ashes were constantly being shoveled from the roofs. The aircraft often landed under difficult circumstances to fetch valuable furnishings, machinery, and goods.

been broken by the air pressure. A short way off, the lava kept running in the same channel as before, vanishing in sea and vapour to the east. It is difficult to describe one's feelings at a sight like this. A once flourishing area had been turned into a desert of pumice and ashes. One could only hope that the rain of cinders would cease and the weather gods come to the help of the islanders by blowing the volcanic debris out to sea.

The days passed, and a real volcanic cone was beginning to form. The salvage operation was going according to schedule; goods of great value were shipped away. The work went on uninterruptedly up to 20 hours a day. It affected everyone's temper; anger flared at the slightest provocation. The pressure on these people was enormous. In addition to everything else, some of them had to witness their houses and possessions disappear under slag and lava. The beautiful one-family homes on the eastern outskirts vanished one after the other. In one place a chimney was jutting up through the pumice, but it soon disappeared, too. Several depressions could be seen where roofs had collapsed, and elsewhere fire was smouldering underneath. Even the hardiest of men came close to sobs watching the abomination of destruction. But they held back their tears and continued their work, salvaging whatever could be salvaged. Bulldozers were beginning to pile up protective barriers between the town and the eruption site, and nobody made a fuss about

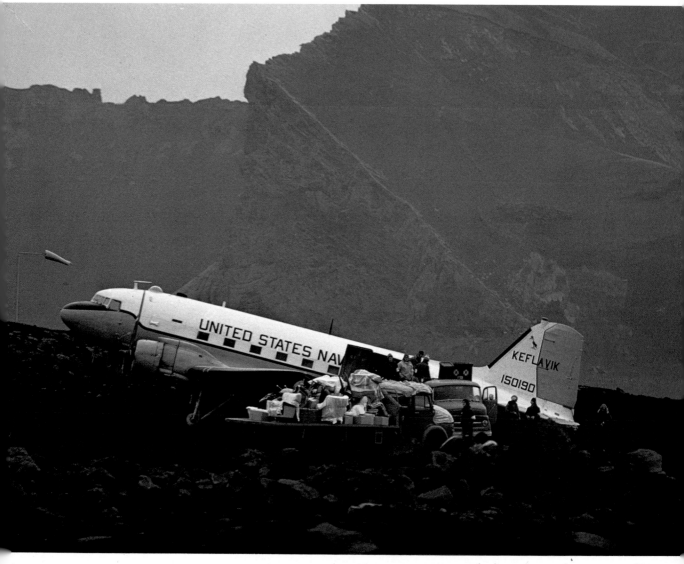

63

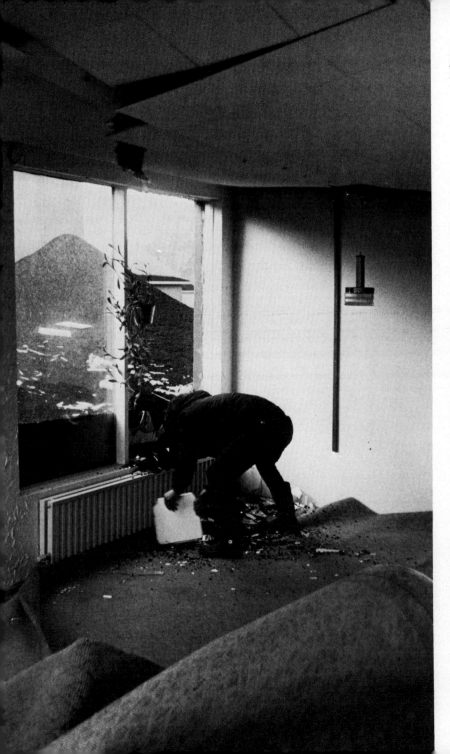

Until the very last moment people tried to save their belongings, even after the roofs of the houses began to cave in (left). And now there was a new mountain which was undeniably beautiful when its slopes glittered in fire at night.

a few houses that were embedded in the bulwarks; they were doomed anyway. The house of the old farmer and those of his six relatives soon vanished from the face of the earth. The new eastern section of the town disappeared completely; those magnificent homes, built at enormous cost by vigorous young men and women, who took pride in making them as handsome as possible, were no longer but a memory. And so it went, day after day. When the force of the eruption seemed to subside, people became hopeful that it would perhaps be over soon, but when its violence increased again such hopes were deflated. While this was happening on the island, new problems began to crop up on the mainland. Permanent homes for the islanders were hard to come by. The people were scattered about the country, but most of them wanted to stay in Reykjavík and other fishing ports nearby. The children had to be placed in schools, and the boats had to find room in other ports. Social difficulties of every kind came to the fore. These had been prosperous people, but they had had to leave their expensive homes and everything that was dear to them; now, suddenly, they were forced to receive everything from others. Actually, the thread of their lives had been partially severed. People used to six or seven rooms had to be content with two or three, the men had to find new jobs, and the children had to get used to new surroundings. Gradually, however, these problems were solved, although there were questions

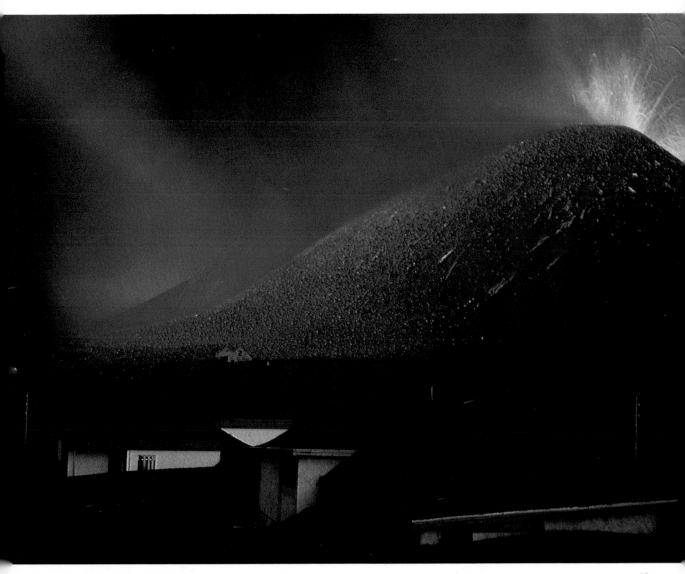

about the wisdom of many decisions. Should an attempt have been made to keep the community together as a whole, instead of scattering people around the country? The islanders themselves would have chosen to remain a „community" as much as possible, but such wishes proved difficult to put into practice. Many ideas were advanced, among them the building of a new town and a new harbour on the southern coast of Iceland, where all the people might be able to live together again. This, it was felt, would alleviate the sorest pain. The mainlanders also had their share of the difficulties; they tried to resolve all the tangles though sometimes it seemed impossible.

It was a balm to frazzled nerves, however, to feel the warm sympathy from the sister nations in Scandinavia, as well as others. Fund-raising was initiated in many countries, and large sums of money were sent to Iceland. People had realized how devastating a blow this natural calamity was for the Icelandic economy — an economy based almost exclusively on fisheries.

Salvage Operations

The days ran into weeks, and the eruption continued. The geologists tried to figure out its nature and how long it would last. It was discovered that the chemical composition of the lava was the same as in Hawaiian eruptions. Accordingly, it could be hoped that the duration of this outburst would be only about a month, similar to the general Hawaiian

pattern. But nobody cared to make any predictions.

At the turn of February the new volcano had acquired a beautiful conic form having reached a height of 540 feet. There was no appreciable reduction in its force. On January 30 it again showered the town with pumice, and this time it contained lots of embers. One more house caught fire, due to the fact that the chimney was filled with red-hot pumice; the fire burst out through the burner. After that, maintenance men were dispatched to inspect houses and clean out chimneys. Others began sweeping the volcanic materials off the roofs, many of which were on the verge of collapse under the weight. One warehouse had already caved in, its walls cracking in the process. Other roofs were reinforced by supporting posts. That day, a large passenger ship also arrived in Vestmannaeyjar, so that people might have the choice of sleeping offshore. Many had found it difficult to sleep in town because of the noise from the eruption site. But people became accustomed to that, too.

The following day the new lava was measured. It proved to be nearly a mile long in a south-north direction along the coast. Triangular in shape, it had a total area of more than half a square mile. That day it was decided that the supervisors of the salvage operation meet daily to coordinate their activities. Iron sheets were now being nailed over the windows of most houses so that the glowing pumice would not have easy

66

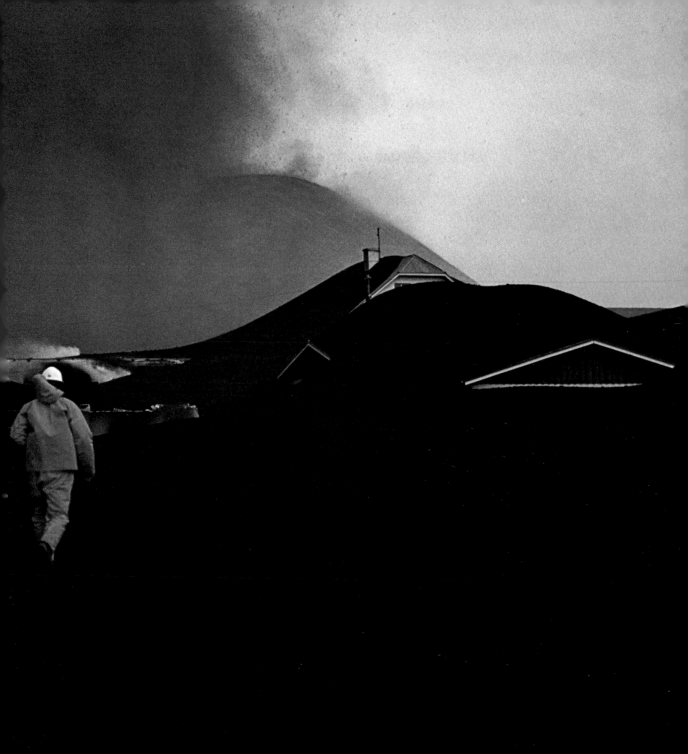

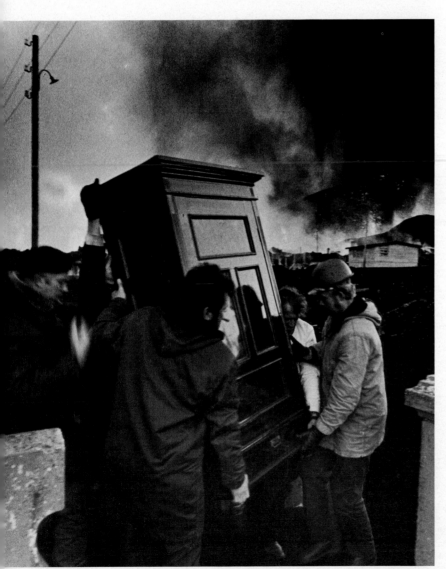

access. The work, executed by more than 70 carpenters who had been flown to the island, was proceeding well. About 100 men were occupied with clearing away the pumice, and some 40 policemen were on duty for general supervisory purposes. That day also, about 40 foreign newsmen arrived on the island; a few had been there earlier. The French television, for instance, had chartered a jet to Heimaey on the first day of the eruption; it had pictures from the island on that evening's news hour.

By this time the volcano had reached an elevation of 600 feet, and the lava kept running. It had now begun to flow on top of the first stream, whose surface had hardened. The scientists continued to observe the eruption very closely, for — as far as is known — this was the first Hawaiian eruption in Iceland since it was settled. The lava was viscous and acidic and somewhat similar to the discharge of the famous Hekla in 1947. But the composition of it was decidedly Hawaiian.

The situation was not equally bad everywhere on the island. In the southern and western sections of town there was, as yet, little pumice, and toward the western coast of the island, where a few farms still hold out, there was only a sprinkling. In some newly cultivated fields one could even see a few fresh green blades of grass. All the sheep from these farms had been taken over to the mainland, and an attempt had also been made to transport the poultry. One farmer sent some 1,100 chickens by boat, but

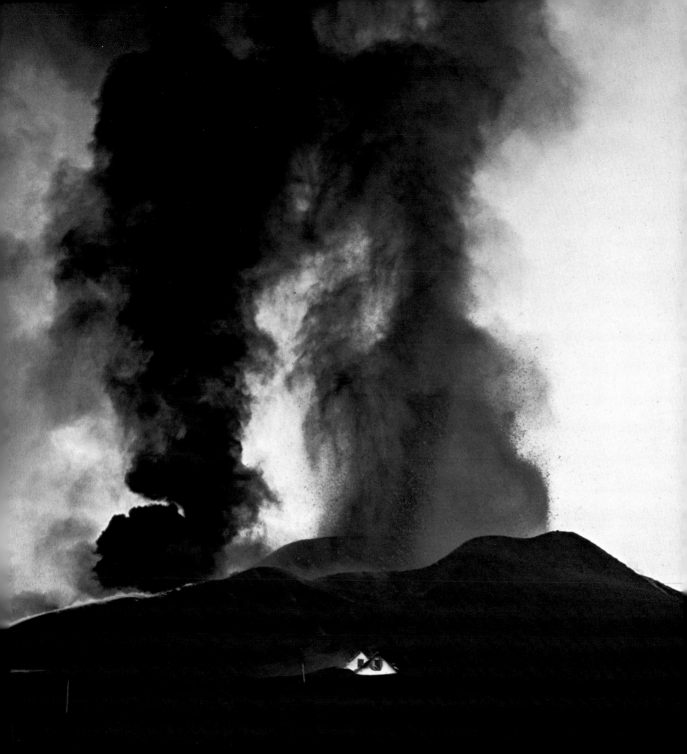

The lava starts flowing towards the entrance of
the harbour, the town's life-nerve. The sea warms
up and steam prevails. The boats appear like
ghost ships when entering the harbour (below).
And the lava flows into the sea. The island has
started growing. Millions of tons of red-hot lava
are to roll into the sea, an amazing sight.

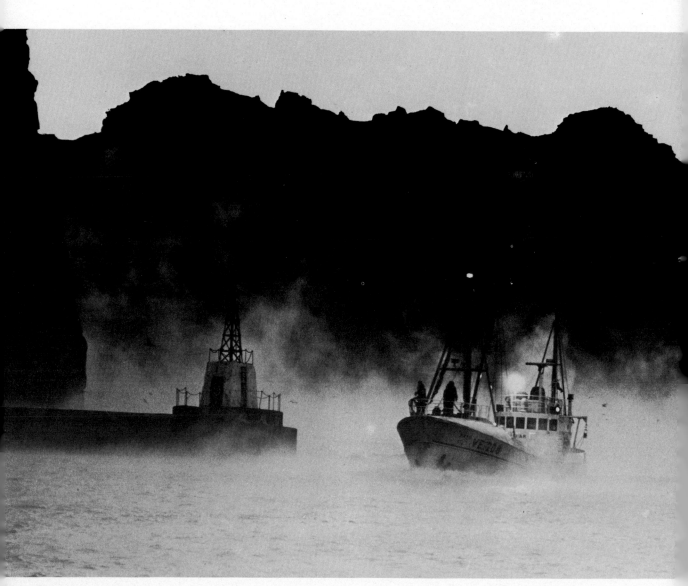

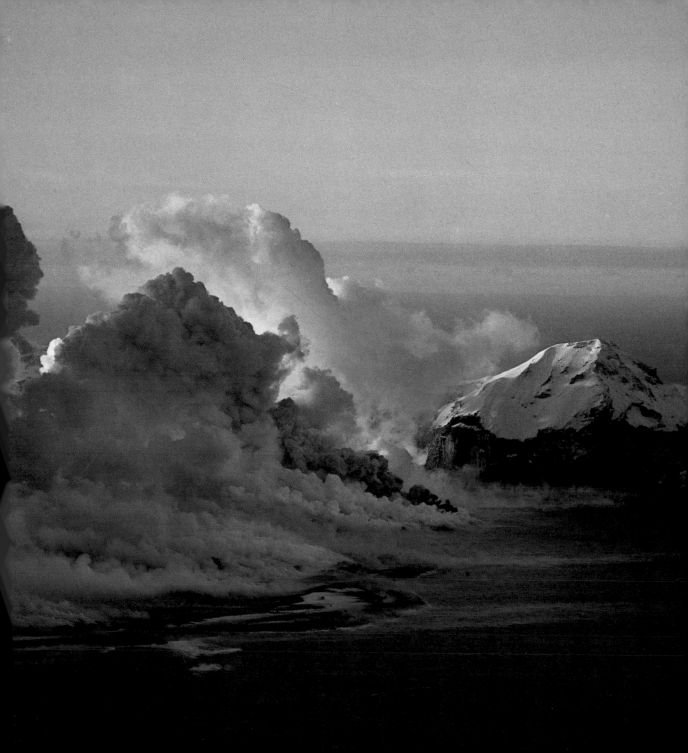

most of them died on the way; only 129 were still alive when the ship reached port. This farmer, however, had kept two roosters and two hens in order to be ready to replenish the stock when the time came. Farther out on the island, where no pumice had yet reached, there is a pretty little inlet, where the islanders sometimes bathe when the weather is clement enough. Here, birds were waddling about the foreshore, and the head of a seal could be seen emerging above the waves; there was much more life than in town. As long as one did not look back toward the eruption site, this spot was like a totally different world.

By January 31, a total of 73 houses had been buried in pumice and 39 had burned. That day, some 12,000 windows had been covered with 95 metric tons of sheet iron. This represented about 85 percent of all the houses in town. There seemed to be no intention of giving up; perhaps life would still triumph. Simultaneously, however, the very same people were preparing to remove equipment worth tens of millions of dollars from the freezing plants. They were not about to take any foolish risks. In addition, furnishings had been carted away from nearly every house in town.

Some inventive fellows thought of placing a television camera on a high cliff overlooking town. Its eye was turned toward the volcano, and unless it was too dark, the people on the mainland could follow the eruption on their home screen whenever the regular programs were not being broadcast. But the camera did not show everything. It missed the men who took a bulldozer to try to find a house that had been buried in the pumice. For some reason, this house had been forgotten during the general removal, and inside it were all the belongings of an entire family. Locating the house presented some difficulties, but once that had been done, the digging began. The bulldozer had to scoop away 15 feet of pumice before the roof came in sight. Then one side of the house was cleared, and, unbelievable as it may sound, all the furnishings were salvaged. Neither did the camera show how a big tractor, with an attached shovel, was hoisted up to the roof of the new hospital in order to speed up the clearance of some 600 metric tons of pumice; there were many other incidents that the camera did not catch.

On February 2, about 100 men of the U. S. Defense Force at Keflavík Airport arrived in Vestmannaeyjar and were immediately put to work clearing volcanic materials off the roofs; they did much good work during the following weeks. More and more people were coming to the island in order to help with the rescue work. Representatives of other nations came there to offer assistance, and newsmen, both foreign and native, were daily visitors. There seemed to be a lull in the eruption, but the wind was extremely irksome. It whirled up the ashes from the ground and the roofs and lashed them into one's face with great ferocity. The finest particles crept under one's collar and seeped down

The liner Gullfoss waits outside the harbour. She is a refuge for the tired rescue workers who must have a rest. An unusual task for this ship, which is always filled with mirth and gayety.

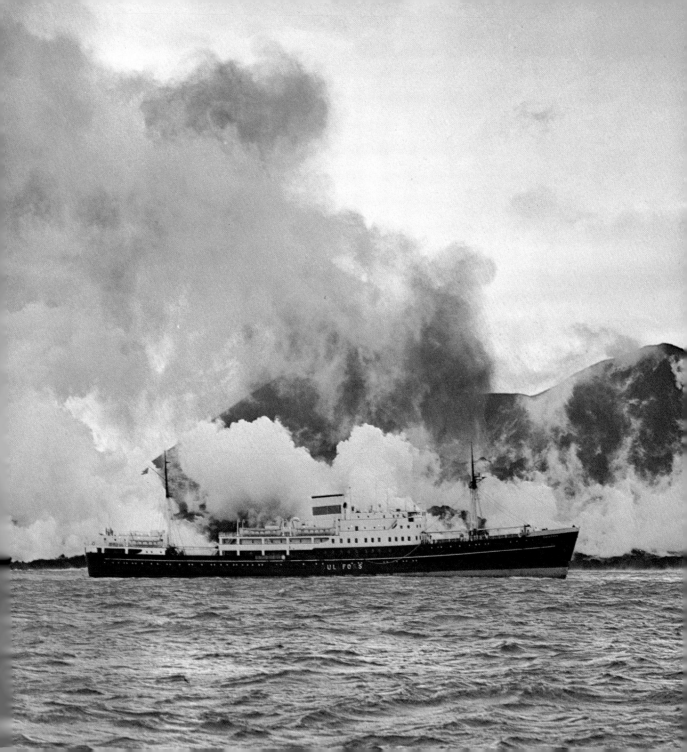

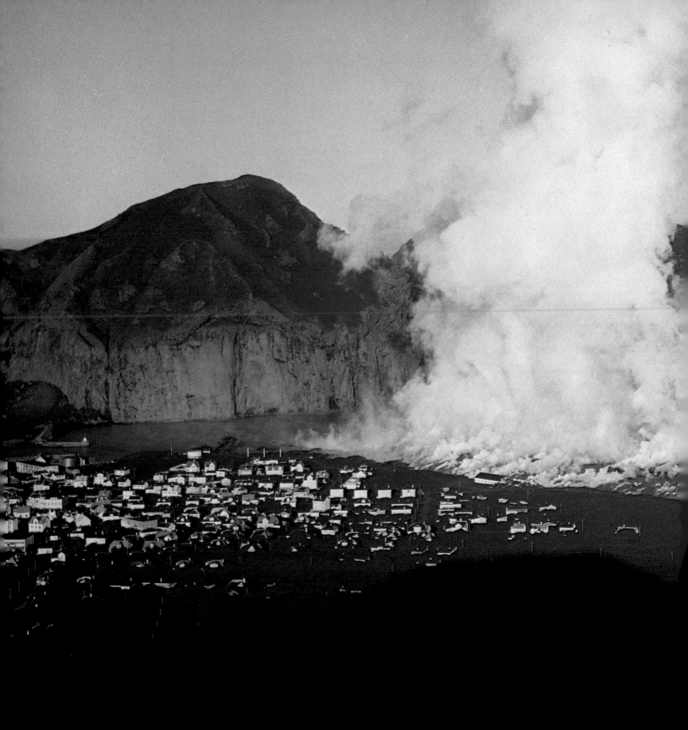

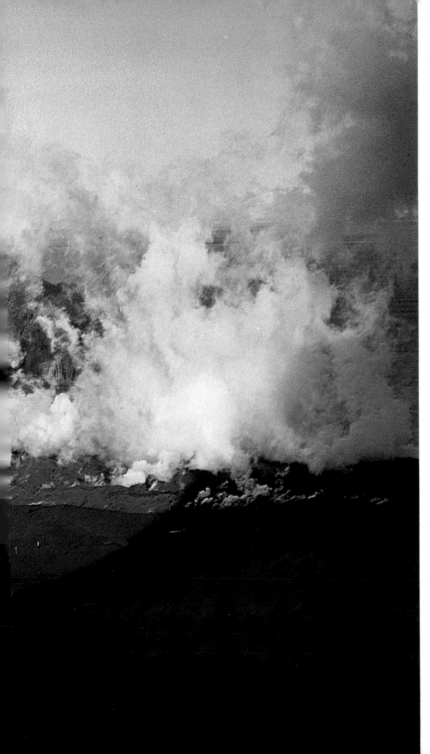

to one's shoes. Worst of all, however, was getting it in the eyes.

General service was good. There was a fine mess hall in one of the freezing plants, where food was served around the clock; the few cooks were close to exhaustion, but the food was excellent. Many islanders, who had emptied their freezers and refrigerators before shipping them to the mainland, had given all the contents to the mess hall. As a result, the tables were laden, day after day, with roast beef, lamb, chicken, pork, and all kinds of other gourmet dishes. No one paid for anything. Strange as it may seem, no money was used on Heimaey during the first days of the eruption; everything was offered free of charge. One shopkeeper opened his store and told people to take whatever they needed. Many workers picked up khakis, windbreakers, work gloves, and other necessities. This good neighbour did not think it was worth the bother to transport his merchandise over to the mainland. He just gave it.

The View from Helgafell

The new volcano was growing higher; it was beginning to rival old Helgafell, which some had, at first, thought responsible for the eruption. But Helgafell maintained its calm and stateliness. East of it lay the fissure, now fallen silent. Small mounds of pumice had piled up over it, and in places where sulphur was predominant the surface took on a yellow-green sheen. The slopes of Helgafell were punctured by countless

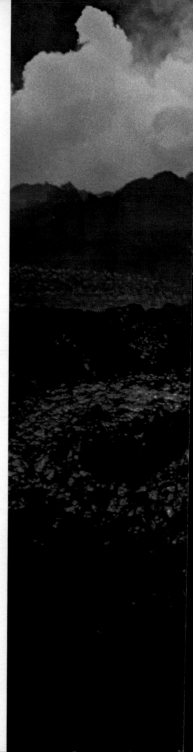

Close to the volcanic area a lava river flows and steadily adds to the lava field to the northeast of the town. Sometimes the lava river moves huge rocks, and the heat is unbearable, being over 1,000° Celcius in the molten lava.

small holes where burning spatters from the new mountain had burrowed through the layer of pumice into the moss beneath. It looked as if many small bombs had been dropped, doing a minimum of damage, but succeeding in igniting the moss, so that smoke frequently rose up from the cavities. Those attentive enough could see many curious things, such as ball-shaped stones which, thrown red-hot from the crater, had revolved in the air with such velocity that they had acquired a global form. The top of Helgafell tempted many photographers, who would sit there for hours on end, taking pictures of the crater which was in full view directly below. The old volcano trembled at the efforts of the new one, and the panoramic points-of-interest indicator at its top could be seen shaking during the worst fits. There was also a good view over the airport, where the traffic of planes, carrying people and cargo, was at a steady peak. This was, in fact, the perfect place from which to look over the landmarks of Heimaey; up there, it became painfully clear how much more the town had suffered from this eruption than other parts of the island. Nowhere else was there so much accumulation of pumice and lava as in and just above the town. One inevitably thought of man's inadequacy when pitted against the forces of nature; the bulldozers piling up ramparts against the advancing lava became ludicrously small in comparison to the volcano. But one's thoughts were also directed to what man can do, if will and courage do not fail, for here, too, one

could see the smoke rising from the fish-meal factory, which had resumed operations after a few days' interval. That smoke was a symbol of optimism.

Once during the early days of the eruption, when newsmen came down from the mountain, they were greeted by a peculiar sight. A young model from a foreign haute couture magazine had planted herself in the churchyard, and scattered about her were suitcases filled with clothes. Dressed in the latest fashion, she had a photographer spinning around her like a satellite, snapping pictures for which the spouting volcano provided the backdrop. No doubt the contrast was striking, but few could appreciate the gimmickry. Some young men wanted to give her a dead cat as a farewell present, just to impress upon her that more was at stake here than a fashion magazine feature. Dead cats were abundant, for many had necessarily been destroyed. Most other animals had been shipped over to the mainland, but many of the cats could not be caught until they were half-dead from hunger and their paws bleeding from stepping over needle-sharp cinders. Representatives of societies for the protection of animals worked diligently saving all living creatures from the island, but birds, such as the snowbunting, were not easily helped. An attempt was made to feed them in places where they converged in large flocks, but the feed was soon buried in pumice and ashes, and the birds became gradually fewer.

The eruption continued, and the weath-

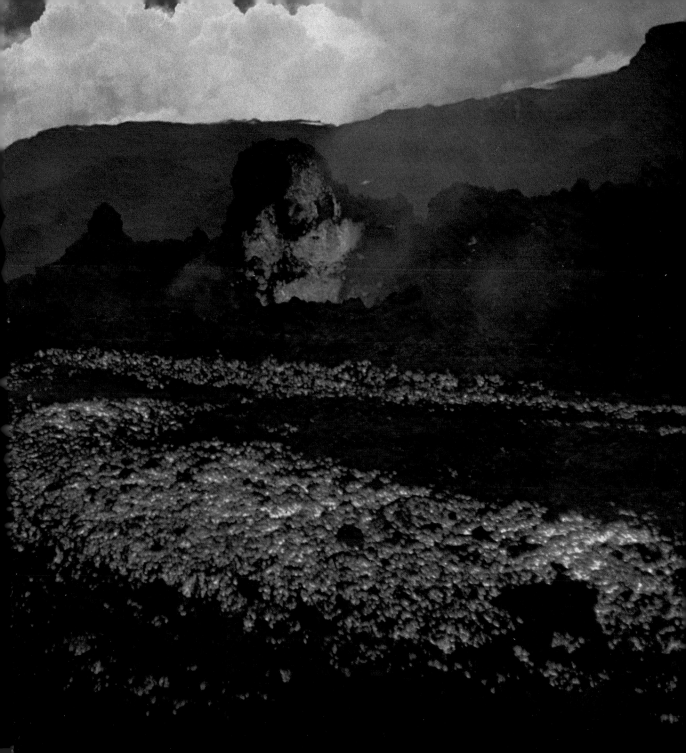

When it snowed, the contrasts were striking
because the snow at once melted on the warm
lava and the new volcano; black and white, fire
and ice. On the picture below, old Helgafell is
to the right, the new volcano to the left.
Compare with the picture on pp. 4–5.

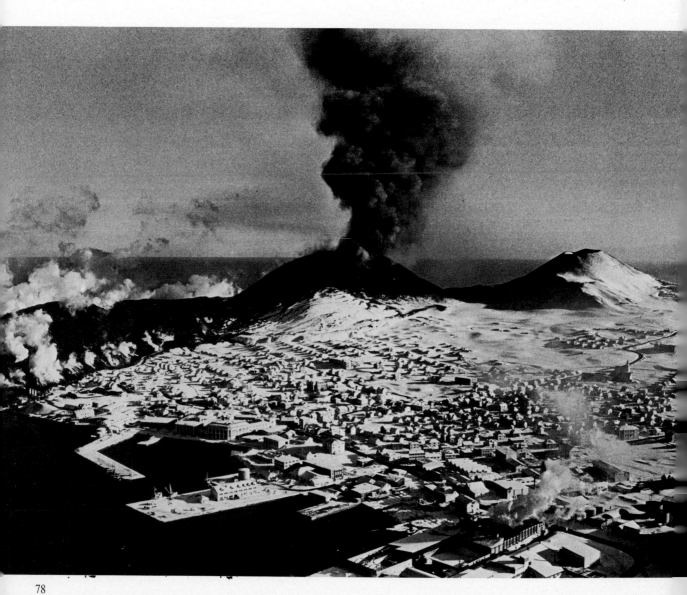

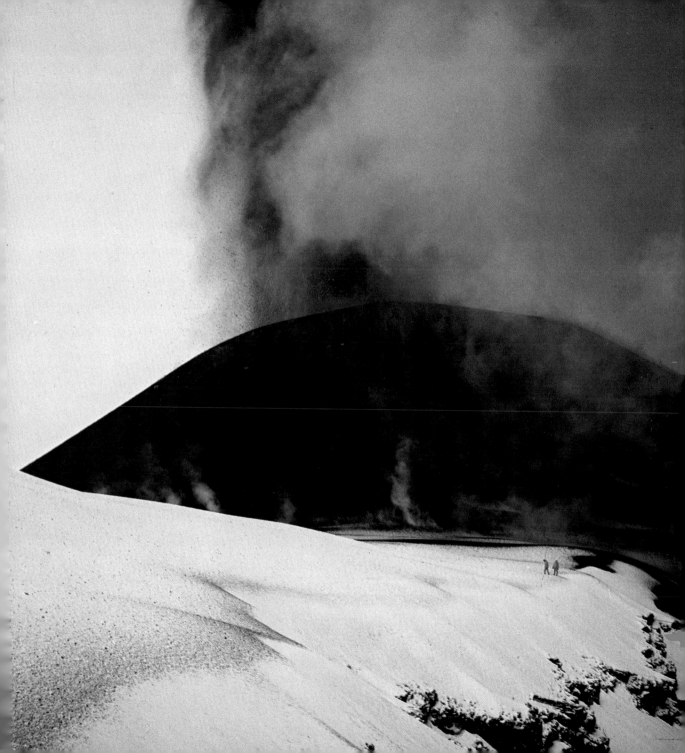

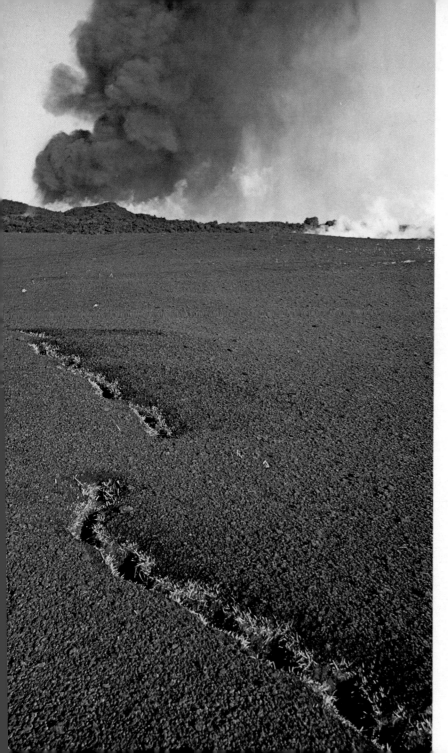

er grew colder. It snowed from time to time, the snow and the pumice covering the island by turns. The layer of pumice thickened steadily, especially when the wind blew from the southeast and carried the material in over the town. One of the major spurts came on February 2. That day it also rained, and the darkness became almost impenetrable; one could hardly see across the street, and the lights practically disappeared in the blackness even though one stood directly beneath the lamppost. In the evening, one more house caught fire. The glowing cinders from the new mountain came trundling down the slopes like a whirling mass of lights and were thrown as far as the centre of town.

The most curious fact about the period of eruption was perhaps the unfaltering continuation of services. The town always had electricity and running water. Automobiles were driven through the streets, planes came and went, and about 500 men were working practically around the clock. Yet all that time, people had a rumbling volcano on their doorstep, spewing fire and brimstone over the town. A widely travelled American newsman who has reported on natural catastrophes and wars alike, said that never before, under similar circumstances, had he been able to live in a comfortable house and enjoy all the amenities of normal conditions. „It's the cosiest disaster I ever observed," he said.

Many more days passed, and the eruption showed little signs of subsiding. There were occasional showers of pumice

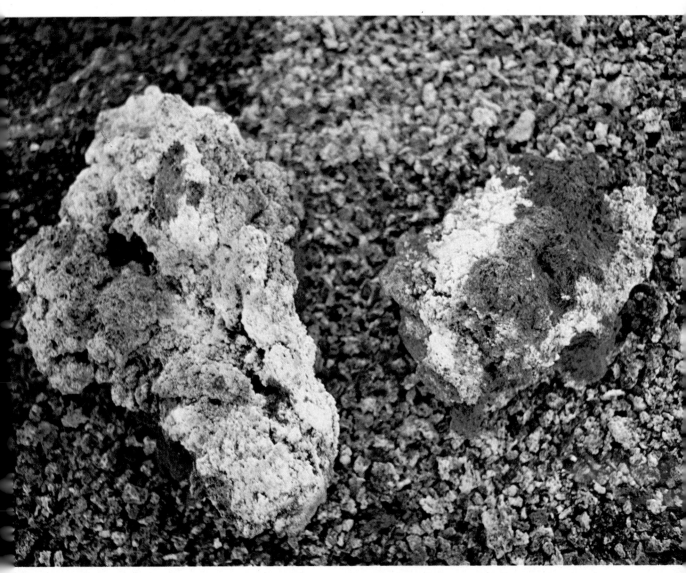

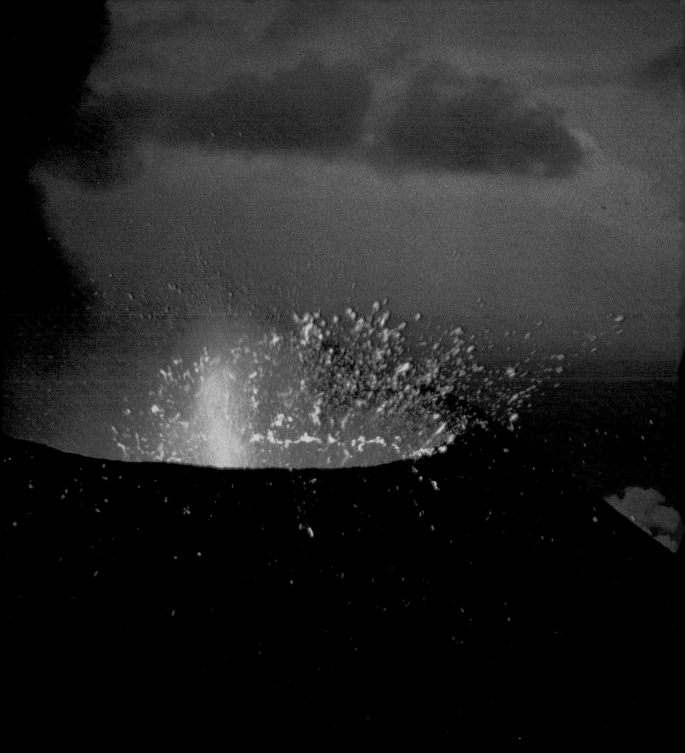

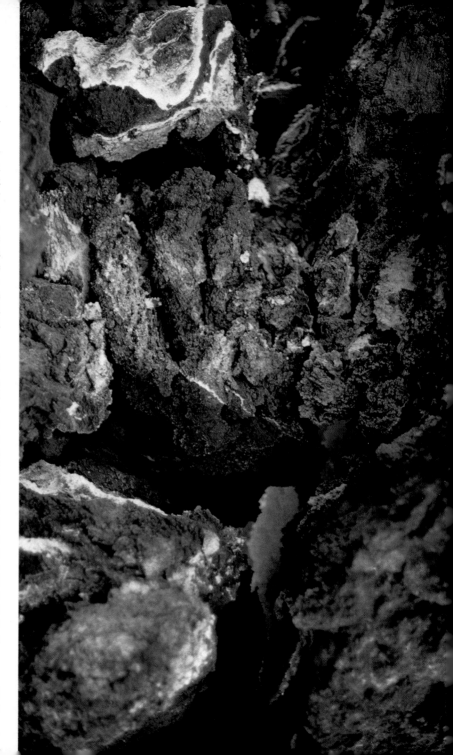

The new volcano is high and has a conical shape. This aerial photograph (left) shows how the splatters squirt over the edges when the lava cauldron boils, while the volcanic activity is at its lowest.
The lava soon cools on the surface when it stops moving, but through the rifts one can see the red-hot lava mass under the thin crust (right).

but, still worse, the lava began to run toward the harbour. This was what people had feared most. Losing a few houses to fire or lava was of little consequence, but if the harbour was closed, the main artery of the community was severed. By February 8, the lava had only 600 more feet to go to block the entrance trench. The water in the harbour became very warm — its temperature was measured at 32 centigrades — and a blanket of vapour spread over it and the vicinity.

Ever since the beginning of the eruption, one of the Icelandic scientists had been very interested in trying to cool the lava by pumping seawater into it. He had previously experimented with this method and shown that it was possible to slow down a lava stream and even to change its course, if its forward edge could be chilled enough. Northeast of the town the lava had built up to a towering brink which threatened to inundate numerous houses. The cooling project was to become a very important part of the salvage operation, and the advance of the lava was, indeed, delayed. It was a gigantic task, especially if one considers that on February 9 it was computed that the quantity of lava discharged from the beginning of the eruption was about 130 million cubic metres; more lava was shown to have flowed out to sea than had been expected.

The Menacing Lava

On February 10 the scientists discovered that the chemical composition of the

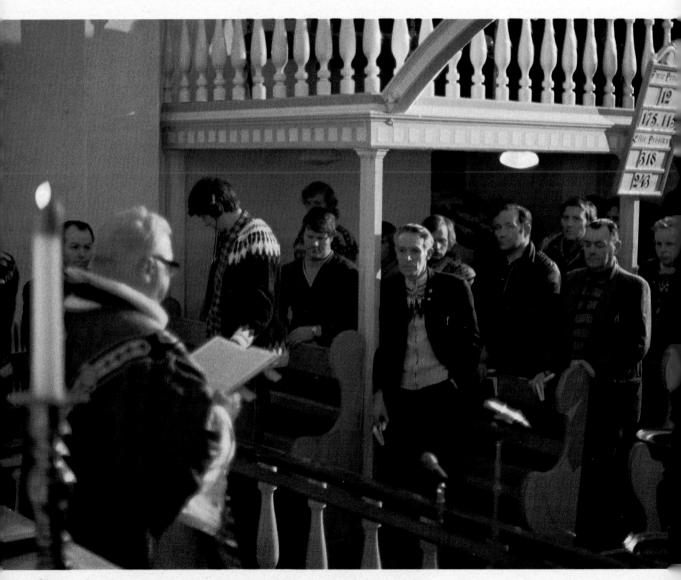

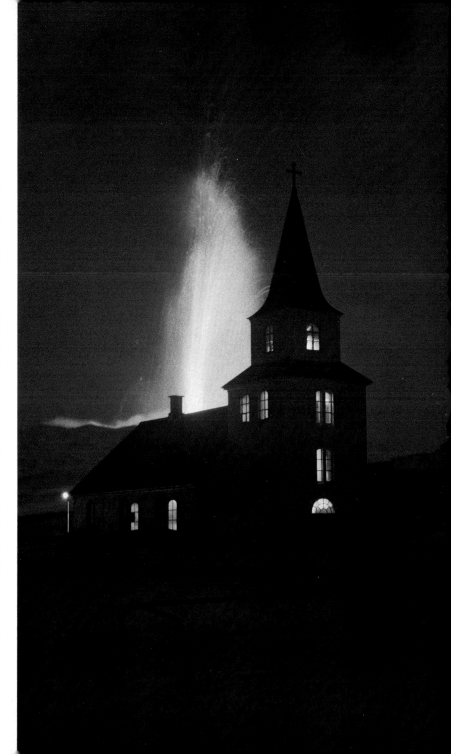

When the volcanic activity was at its height, the parson announced a service in the church one evening, and it was filled with dead-tired rescue workers (opposite). The atmosphere was peculiar, hymn singing with the roar of the volcano as a kind of accompaniment.

lava had changed from what it had been in the beginning. The volcanic rock was no longer Hawaiian but more like that of Surtsey. That seemed to kill all hopes that this outburst would last only a short time. It was recalled that the Surtsey eruption had continued for more than three years and had flared up in many places. It was also becoming increasingly clear that the edge of the lava was pushing forward under its own weight. This menacing brink above the town had grown about 120 feet high, much taller than most houses in town, especially the nearest ones. The pressure of this massive pile of rock squeezed out the molten lava underneath, causing it to dart out suddenly and unpredictably — as often as not in the direction of the town. The main flow was still northeastward into the sea, where it did no harm. As no current was perceptible on the surface, it was concluded that the lava was running through underground channels.

One more problem was now encountered. The weather had grown colder, and the water that had been left in the heating systems, when people abandoned their homes, was beginning to freeze. Pipes inside walls as well as radiators burst and caused much damage to numerous interiors. Cellars filled with water, and walls were ruined by the cracking pipes. A host of salvage workers tried to save what could be saved and, indeed, prevented the ruination of many buildings.

For some time, the idea of trying to change the course of the lava by blasting new channels for it was seriously

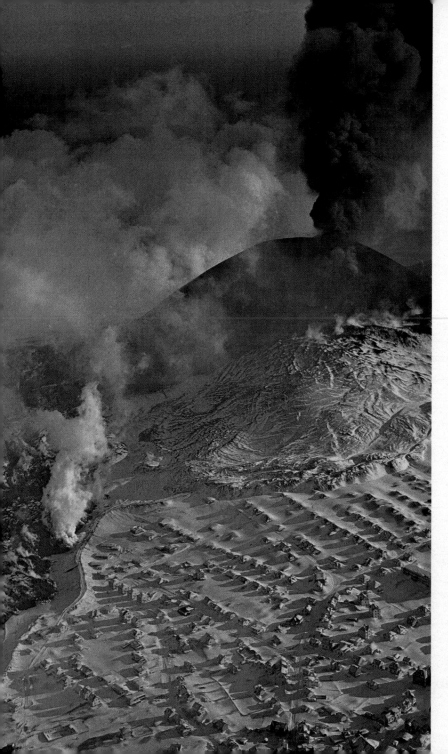

The lava continues to stretch itself over the town, and the protective embankments are of little avail, when the thrust is at its strongest. Off and on, a thin cover of snow lay over the town, since this was in mid-winter, but as a rule the pitch-black colour of the pumice dominated.

pondered. American demolition experts were invited to Vestmannaeyjar and small plastic bombs were shipped over for experimentation. The issue was discussed from every possible angle; whether or not to use planes to drop the bombs, and how they could be used to greatest advantage. After extensive observations, however, the conclusion was reached that because the volcano was so close to the town, the use of explosives would be too risky. No one could predict what the consequences might be. For all they knew, such a step might even quicken the progress of the lava toward the town.

On February 12 all boats were ordered out of the Vestmannaeyjar harbour because the lava had advanced so much the previous night that the port was in danger of closing. Mountainous heaps of pumice had formed out on the lava tract; from their tops was an excellent view over the new lava. These heaps were constantly moving, carried along with the stream.

The lava running toward the harbour finally severed the electric cable to the island. Then it came in handy to have the old diesel plant in workable condition. It could produce sufficient electricity for the whole town. The lava also cut one of the submarine water mains, but the other had apparently been covered with enough pumice to enable it to withstand the weight of the more solid lava. So, water and electricity were still adequate, and people were not yet about to surrender.

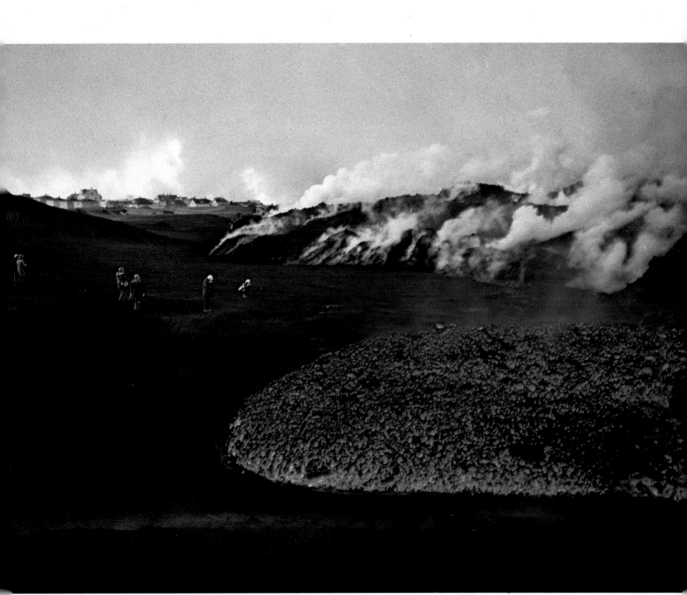

Then the volcanic gas began to flow. The night before February 15, it was confirmed that gas had found its way into several houses. The phenomenon was known from the 1947 eruption of Hekla, when it was found in depressions and hollows; it killed several sheep at the time. This gas is heavy and stays close to the ground, but where it gains access to closed cellars or houses, it can pile up and saturate the air. It can then become explosive. The gas can kill people in a few minutes, and before it was discovered indoors, several men who had walked over the new lava had been affected by it. They got a headache and became very weak, but recovered quickly when they breathed better air. One house had already exploded from this gas.

Another Pompeii?

On the evening the chemists were analyzing the gas, the first social gathering since the beginning of the eruption was held in Vestmannaeyjar. It was the kind of mid-winter celebration Icelanders call thorrablót. On such occasions, great quantities of sour food, pickled since early autumn, is served. There was plenty of such food in the islands. A few young men formed a committee and prepared the affair in the largest hall in town. They invited everybody who happened to be on the island, and most of these attended. There were close to 500 men, but only eight women, and the sounds of admiration emitted by the horde of males as the women made their entrance may be easily imagined. The party included nearly 400 Icelanders and about 100 Americans of the Defense Force. It was a tired and stubbly group of men, but that night they managed to forget what was happening outside the walls of the hall. They ate and sang, watched homemade entertainment numbers, as well as a Western. But what most pleased them, perhaps, were the telegrams they received — cabled thanks for a job well done. One of the telegrams was from four well-known elderly islanders, who happened to be all lying in the same hospital in Reykjavík. It said, „We thank all of you for your great work for the welfare of our island and of the whole nation. Will all return in the spring, when the puffin comes back home. Be well, skál, and best regards." One of the four was the old farmer who had lost everything he had called his. When the gathering was over, around 1:00 a.m., the men dispersed into the darkness. In the morning, after a few hours of sleep, they would resume their salvage work. Some ashes were falling, and the gas was increasing.

Still more days passed, and the eruption continued. The tract of lava grew larger and higher every day. The cooling project proceeded as planned, appreciably slowing the flow toward the town. A 90-foot high edge piled up, but the main part of the lava ran northeastward into the sea. The entrance to the harbour was somewhat narrowed, the lava finally reached one of the breakwaters. At that point it was decided no longer to risk the equipment of the processing plants,

The lava now and again assaulted the town and crushed both dwelling-houses and larger edifices. As a rule the houses went up in flames as they first touched this red-hot lava mass, but sometimes they had not been fully burned down when they disappeared under the lava.

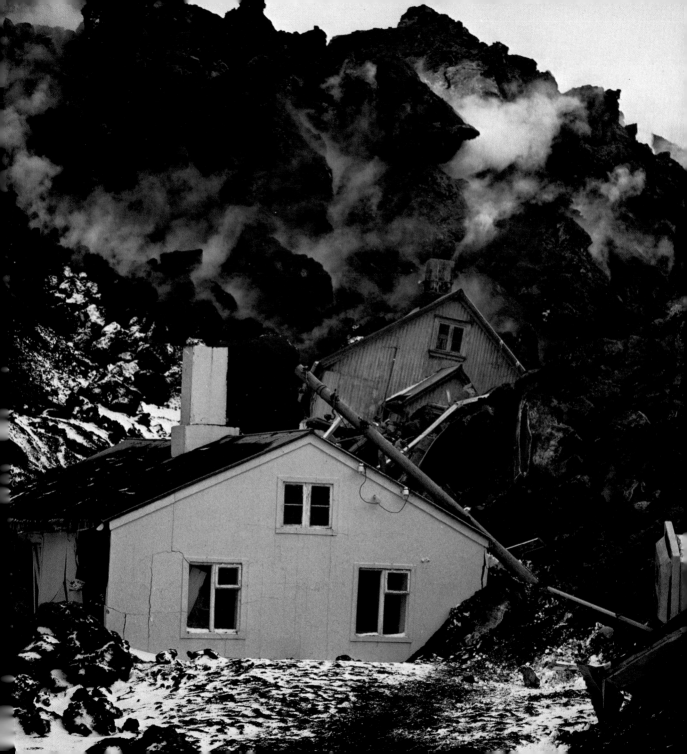

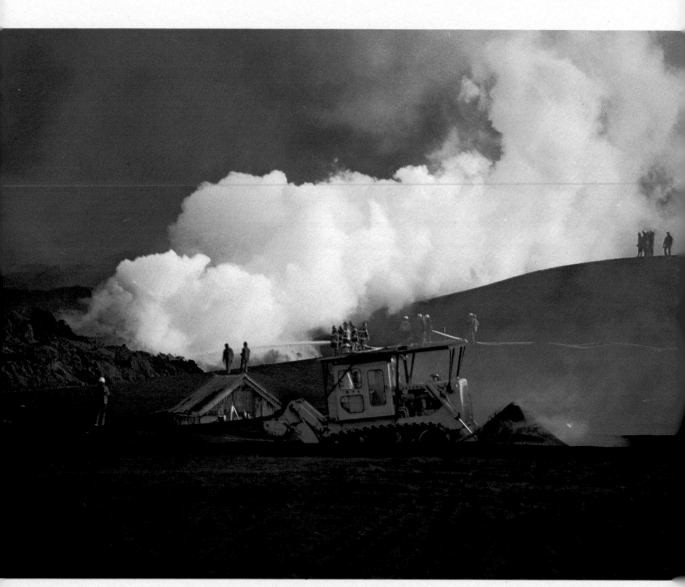

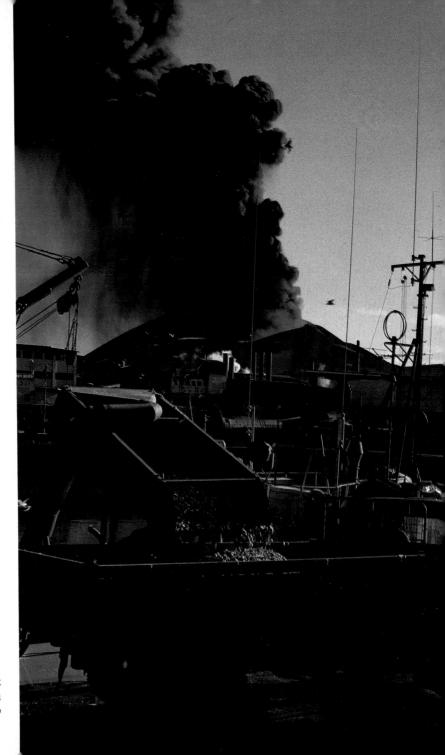

While nature played havoc with the island, the fishermen landed their capelin catch undaunted, and it was processed under the worst possible circumstances, in constant danger. No one wanted to give up until it came to the pinch (right).

which was worth millions of dollars. The U. S. government made available two large cargo craft which could land at the island's airport, and these, along with Icelandic planes, began to carry off machinery. Every ton of this equipment was valued at $ 20,000. The transportation, involving hundreds of tons, was completed without difficulties. At the same time, machinery and tools from other establishments, such as repair shops, furniture workshops, and stores, were shipped away; by this time, most residences on the island had been practically emptied. One man was seriously injured during these operations, and another had been hurt shortly before, when trying to safe the roof of a house. But no one had been killed.

Then, one day, the western side of the new volcano crumbled. It was the side facing the town. Millions of tons of slag and pumice slid down in an avalanche, but was stopped by one of the protective barriers. The volcanic discharge burying the easternmost houses had reached a thickness of 120 feet. When the volcano crumbled, a great heap of pumice began moving on top of the lava tract, progressing up to 100 feet a day toward the entrance of the harbour. No one knew where it would stop.

While this was happening in Vestmannaeyjar, people on the mainland were busy trying to find permanent places for the refugees. It was decided that prefabricated homes be purchased from Norway and other countries in order to reduce the shortage of housing. They would be located in fishing ports on the southern shore. Many islanders were still living in summer cottages and apartments of relatives and friends.

Their boats, however, continued fishing and, as usual, fishing well; the capelin season had never been better. The fish-meal factory on Heimaey had decided to process the catch; it was working around the clock at top capacity. Still, people kept wondering if the time had come to put the period after the story of Vestmannaeyjar. Nobody wanted to, at least not publicly. A great deal of money was being spent on the salvage operation. Some said it was a total waste, but the majority felt that everything possible should be done to save the town.

The gas was now becoming a serious problem. People were getting sick, and large parts of the town had to be closed to all traffic. Bulldozers pushed together big mounds of pumice in the streets in these sections, so that no automobile could drive through. People were apt to become ill quite suddenly; they became very weak, lost consciousness, and were totally helpless. The telephone office and the navigational radio station, as well as the centre of the salvage operation, had to be moved to higher ground. Around the middle of March, the lava also became much more aggressive. Twelve new one-family houses disappeared under it in one day. More and more emphasis was being placed on the cooling project. Water pipes were laid along the entire edge of the lava facing the town, and potent machinery, including ships equipped with high-pressure pumps, was secured to sprinkle the lava day and night. The edge at the mouth of the harbour was a particular target for these powerful jets of cold sea.

The crew of workers on the island was reduced; only about 300 were left. Inflatable rubber rafts were kept ready on shore in case an emergency evacuation became necessary and the harbour was blocked. Lava kept constantly oozing out of the crater, and from time to time the town was showered with ashes. In more than one case, women had come back to the island to clean their houses before they were engulfed by the lava. Their homes were to be immaculate to the end. One man raised the flag at half mast when the flow reached the gable of his home. He was saying farewell to a close friend.

The land around the town had acquired a new aspect, totally unrecognizable. Where before there had been green fields, handsome houses, and gardens, were now mountains and hills, all formed in a mere two months. The town was bordered on two sides by towering heaps of slag and lava, higher by far than the tallest houses, and getting bigger by the day. It was a nightmare of a reality.

Many asked, „Are the Vestmannaeyjar to become another Pompeii?" That would, indeed, be a deplorable fate for one of the most prosperous communities in Iceland.

92

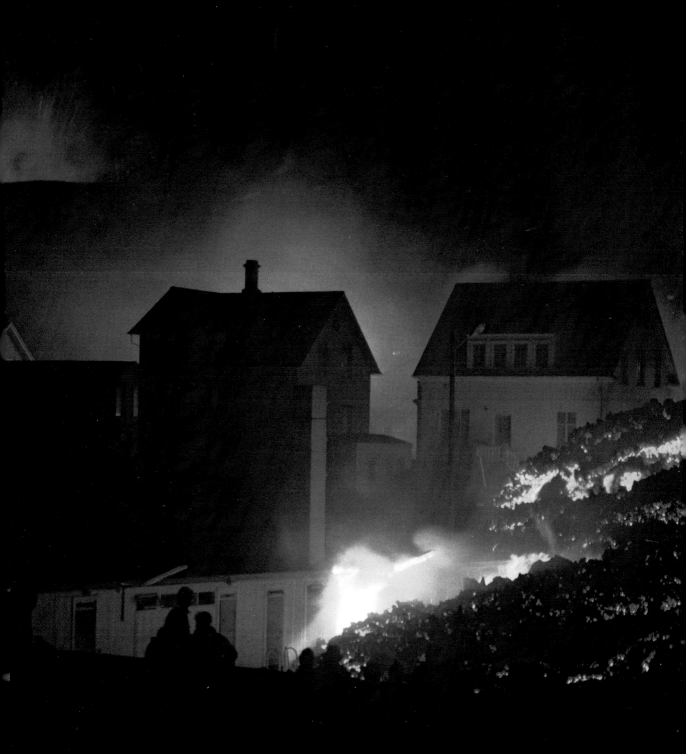

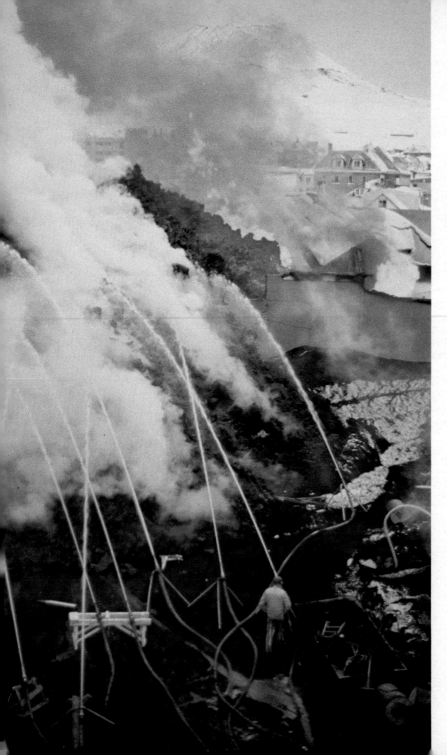

As the days passed the lava swallowed dozens of new houses. It stretched itself into the centre of town, and the danger that it may block the harbour entrance and fill the harbour will be imminent as long as the eruption lasts. The pumping of seawater in order to cool the lava current is going on day and night without interruption. No stone is left unturned in the endeavours to save the harbour, the very life-nerve of this community. The inhabitants of Vestmannaeyjar are not going to give up until all hope is futile and in vain. They wait in suspense for the day when they can return to their island. Whether the eruption will last half a year or four years, nobody knows — and whether anything will be left of this prosperous community when the catastrophe at last comes to a halt, no one knows either. We can only wait and hope — cling to the hope as long as it is there. There is nothing else we can do.

The lava has pressed forward into the centre of town and conquered many of the most important means of production, the freezing plants, the power station, etc., and is only a stone's throw from the harbour.

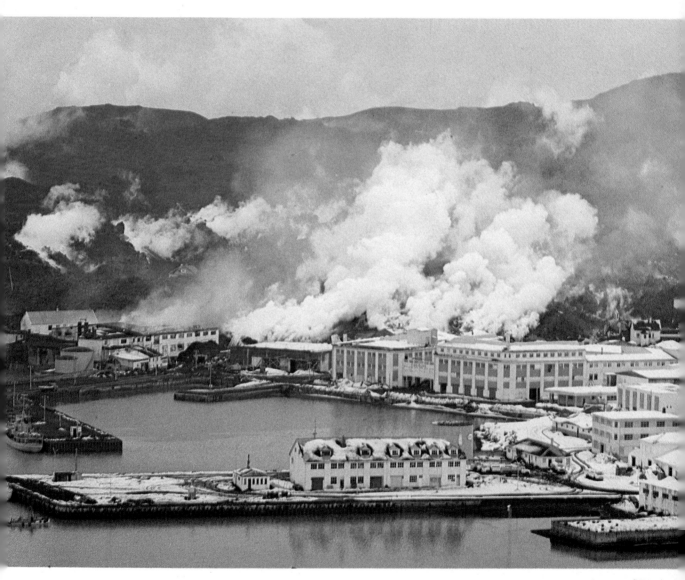

Will the lava block the entrance to the harbour or will the people of Vestmannaeyjar retain their life-nerve? The question is not, how many houses will go under the lava, but whether the harbour will be usable after this battle is over. The channel has become very narrow. The lava must not advance much further. Compare this photo with the one on page 28.

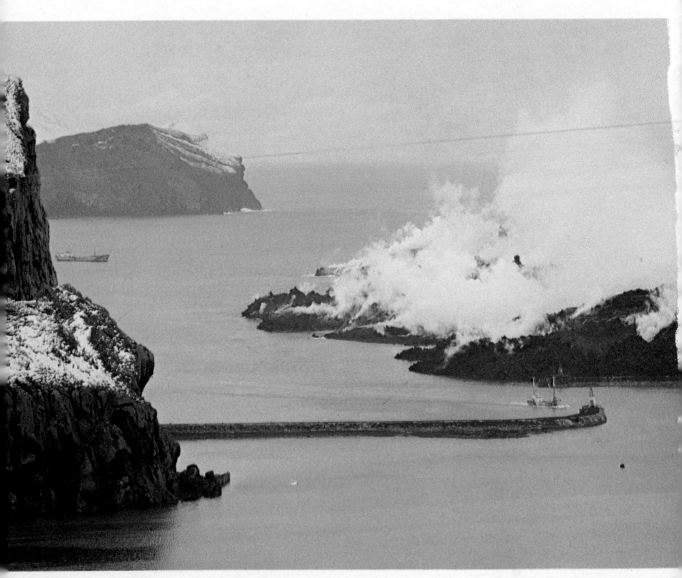

Text:
Árni Gunnarsson

Translation:
May and Hallberg Hallmundsson

Lay-out:
AUGLÝSINGASTOFAN H.F., Gísli B. Björnsson

Designer:
Fanney Valgardsdóttir

Publisher:
ICELAND REVIEW©, 1973,
Reykjavik, Iceland

Printed in The Netherlands by Boom-Ruygrok

ICELAND REVIEW BOOKS.
Previously published in this series:
ICELAND – the Unspoiled Land

Photos:

Björn Rúriksson	Page	65
Bragi Gudmundsson		42, 61, 64
Gardar Pálsson		9
Gudjón Eggertsson		70
Gudmundur Ingólfsson		73
Gunnar Hannesson		7, 8, 13, 20, 26, 28, 32, 33, 46, 59, 86
Helgi Torfason		87
Kristinn Benediktsson		44, 56
Kristinn Helgason		82
Kristján P. Gudnason		89, 93
Kristjón Haraldsson		40
Leifur Thorsteinsson		31
Mats Wibe Lund		5
Owen Franken		62, 63
Rafn Hafnfjörd		19, 71, 90
Sigurdur Thórarinsson		77, Back Cover
Sigurgeir Jónasson		3, 10, 11, 14, 15, 17, 18, 22, 23, 25, 27, 43, 45, 50, 57, 67, 78, 79, 80, 81, 83, 84, 85, 91, 94, 95, 96
Sigurgeir Sigurjónsson		Front Cover, 37, 49, 53, 54, 55, 68
Sveinn Thormódsson		39, 41
Wedigo Ferchland		38, 51
Ævar Jóhannesson		34, 69, 74

CONTRIBUTORS

Matthew S. Austin, MD
Assistant Professor
Department of Orthopaedic Surgery
Thomas Jefferson University/
   Rothman Institute
Philadelphia, Pennsylvania

David Backstein, MD, MEd, FRCSC
Hip and Knee Reconstruction
Division of Orthopaedic Surgery
Mt. Sinai Hospital
University of Toronto
Toronto, Ontario, Canada

Hari P. Bezwada, MD
Associate Professor
Booth Bartolozzi Balderston Orthopaedics
Pennsylvania Hospital
Philadelphia, Pennsylvania

Craig J. Della Valle, MD
Associate Professor of Orthopaedics
Director, Adult Reconstructive Fellowship
Rush University Medical Center
Chicago, Illinois

Nitin Goyal, MD
Chief Resident
Department of Orthopaedic Surgery
Thomas Jefferson University Hospital
Philadelphia, Pennsylvania

Atul F. Kamath, MD
Clinical Instructor
Department of Orthopaedic Surgery
University of Pennsylvania
Philadelphia, Pennsylvania

Gregg R. Klein, MD
Attending Orthopaedic Surgeon
Department of Orthopaedic Surgery
Hackensack University Medical Center
Hackensack, New Jersey

Harlan B. Levine, MD
Attending Orthopaedic Surgeon
Department of Orthopaedic Surgery
Hackensack University Medical Center
Hackensack, New Jersey

Jess H. Lonner, MD
Attending Orthopaedic Surgeon
Rothman Institute at Bryn Mawr Hospital
Associate Professor of Orthopaedic Surgery
Thomas Jefferson University
Philadelphia, Pennsylvania

Wadih Y. Matar, MD, MSc, FRCSC
Orthopaedic Surgeon, Adult Reconstruction
Division of Orthopaedic Surgery
CSSS de Gatineau – Hull Hospital
Gatineau, Quebec, Canada

R. Michael Meneghini, MD
Assistant Professor of Clinical Orthopaedic
   Surgery
Department of Orthopaedic Surgery
Indiana Clinic
Indiana University School of Medicine
Indianapolis, Indiana

Michael Todd Newman, MD
Adult Reconstruction Fellow
Booth Bartolozzi Balderston Orthopaedics
Pennsylvania Hospital
Philadelphia, Pennsylvania

Alvin Ong, MD
Orthopaedic Surgeon
Rothman Institute
Egg Harbor Township, New Jersey

Fabio Orozco, MD
Orthopaedic Surgeon
Rothman Institute
Egg Harbor Township, New Jersey

CONTRIBUTORS (CONT.)

Javad Parvizi, MD, FRCS
Professor of Orthopaedic Surgery
Thomas Jefferson University
Philadelphia, Pennsylvania

James J. Purtill, MD
Assistant Professor
Thomas Jefferson University/
  Rothman Institute
Philadelphia, Pennsylvania

Gordon H. Stock, MD
Adult Reconstruction Fellow
Department of Orthopaedic Surgery
Thomas Jefferson University Hospital/
  Rothman Institute
Philadelphia, Pennsylvania

Emmanuel Thienpont, MD, MBA
Department of Orthopaedic Surgery
University Hospital Saint Luc
Brussels, Belgium

Principles and Techniques In Revision Total Knee Arthroplasty

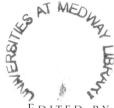

Edited by
Javad Parvizi, MD, FRCS
Professor of Orthopaedic Surgery
Thomas Jefferson University
Philadelphia, Pennsylvania

Series Editor
Henry D. Clarke, MD
Consultant, Department of Orthopedic Surgery
Associate Professor of Orthopedic Surgery, College of Medicine
Mayo Clinic
Phoenix, Arizona

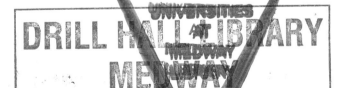

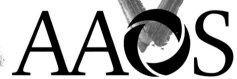

AAOS
American Academy of Orthopaedic Surgeons

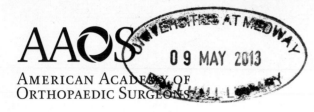

Revision Total Knee Arthroplasty

Published 2012 by the
American Academy of Orthopaedic Surgeons
6300 North River Road
Rosemont, IL 60018

The material presented in *Revision Total Knee Arthroplasty* has been made available by the American Academy of Orthopaedic Surgeons for educational purposes only. This material is not intended to present the only, or necessarily best, methods or procedures for the medical situations discussed, but rather is intended to represent an approach, view, statement, or opinion of the author(s) or producer(s), which may be helpful to others who face similar situations.

Some drugs or medical devices demonstrated in Academy courses or described in Academy print or electronic publications have not been cleared by the Food and Drug Administration (FDA) or have been cleared for specific uses only. The FDA has stated that it is the responsibility of the physician to determine the FDA clearance status of each drug or device he or she wishes to use in clinical practice.

Furthermore, any statements about commercial products are solely the opinion(s) of the author(s) and do not represent an Academy endorsement or evaluation of these products. These statements may not be used in advertising or for any commercial purpose.

Copyright 2012
by the American Academy of Orthopaedic Surgeons

ISBN
978-0-89203-842-8
Printed in the USA

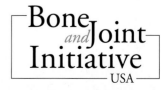

CONTENTS

PREFACE   vii

1   BASIC PRINCIPLES OF REVISION TOTAL KNEE
ARTHROPLASTY   1

Michael Todd Newman, MD
Hari P. Bezwada, MD

2   PREOPERATIVE PLANNING FOR REVISION
TOTAL KNEE ARTHROPLASTY   11

Wadih Y. Matar, MD, MSc, FRCSC

3   EXPOSURE FOR REVISION TOTAL KNEE
ARTHROPLASTY   17

Craig J. Della Valle, MD

4   PROSTHESIS SELECTION: CHOOSING THE
RIGHT TYPE OF CONSTRAINT   29

Emmanuel Thienpont, MD, MBA

5   PERIPROSTHETIC KNEE INFECTIONS:
CONTRIBUTING FACTORS   41

Nitin Goyal, MD
James J. Purtill, MD

6   MANAGEMENT OF BONE LOSS IN REVISION
TOTAL KNEE ARTHROPLASTY   49

Gordon H. Stock, MD
Matthew S. Austin, MD
R. Michael Meneghini, MD

7   MANAGEMENT OF EXTENSOR MECHANISM
DISRUPTION AFTER TOTAL KNEE
ARTHROPLASTY   63

Fabio Orozco, MD
Alvin Ong, MD

8   REVISION TOTAL KNEE ARTHROPLASTY
FOR INFECTION   77

Atul F. Kamath, MD
Jess H. Lonner, MD

9   REVISION TOTAL KNEE ARTHROPLASTY FOR
PERIPROSTHETIC FRACTURE   89

David Backstein, MD, MEd, FRCSC

10   REVISION TOTAL KNEE ARTHROPLASTY
FOR INSTABILITY   103

Gregg R. Klein, MD
Harlan B. Levine, MD

PREFACE

Total knee arthroplasty (TKA) is one of the most successful orthopaedic surgical procedures ever developed. This procedure has alleviated pain and suffering and afforded function in many thousands of patients. In a minority of patients, however, early or late failure occurs, necessitating revision arthroplasty.

Revision Total Knee Arthroplasty is written by recognized world authorities in the field of revision TKA. The information presented here is based on available evidence regarding management of failed TKA. The chapters cover both common and uncommon etiologies of failure and options for management. The text is richly illustrated and offers detailed, step-by-step descriptions of the surgical management for each condition. The goal of this monograph is to provide useful and practical guidance to the orthopaedic surgeon who treats these patients.

I am most grateful to the authors for sharing their wisdom and surgical expertise. I also offer sincere gratitude to Laurie Braun, managing editor at the American Academy of Orthopaedic Surgeons (AAOS), for her leadership in executing this assignment and her extremely useful editorial corrections and suggestions that enhanced the quality of this work immensely. Finally, I would like to thank the Publications Department at the AAOS for making this important publication a reality.

I hope that you will find this publication useful in restoring function to your patients.

Javad Parvizi, MD, FRCS
Editor

CHAPTER 1

BASIC PRINCIPLES OF REVISION TOTAL KNEE ARTHROPLASTY

MICHAEL TODD NEWMAN, MD

HARI P. BEZWADA, MD

INTRODUCTION

Revision total knee arthroplasty (TKA) presents a true challenge for both the general orthopaedist and the fellowship-trained adult reconstruction surgeon. The number of primary TKAs performed in the United States continues to rise as the population ages and is due to the unparalleled surgical success of this procedure in terms of pain relief and increased patient function. The newer generation implants that are used today have increased longevity; however, the orthopaedic community is beginning to encounter with greater frequency those patients who underwent primary TKAs 15 to 20 years ago. From 1990 to 2002, the number of primary and revision TKAs each increased by more than 200%.[1] The number of revision TKAs is expected to rise substantially over the next 20 years; recent estimates anticipate a greater than 600% increase, to 268,000 procedures per year.[2] This presents quite a challenge to the healthcare system with respect to workload and financial burden, as revision surgery has been estimated to cost $15,000 to $40,000 per patient.[1]

Before performing a revision TKA, a thorough evaluation is essential to determine the reason for failure (**Figures 1** and **2**). This begins with a complete history and physical examination, focusing on the main symptoms. The causes of most primary TKA failures fall into several broad categories, including infection, instability, and loosening.[3] The initial evaluation must include a detailed search for these etiologies. For instance, a history of fevers, nausea, vomiting, or night sweats usually indicates infection. Physical examination can usually easily identify instability or patellar maltracking. Radiographs are essential and can indicate polyethylene wear or osteolysis. Often, however, the reason for failure is elusive and requires a more complete workup, including aspiration, laboratory testing (erythrocyte sedimentation rate [ESR] and C-reactive protein [CRP] level), fluoroscopic evaluation or bone scanning, and either white blood cell count tagged to evaluate for infection or standard nuclear scanning to evaluate for occult loosening. Despite an exhaustive workup, however, the reason for failure may not be identified or complex regional pain syndrome may have developed. In these instances, it is often best to avoid advising revision surgery because results after revision TKA are poor when the surgery is performed for no identified reason.[4]

Once a definitive etiology of failure has been determined and surgery is deemed the most appropriate treatment option, the operating surgeon must keep in mind several important principles. Most of these principles can be addressed with exhaustive preoperative planning. During this exercise, the surgeon can contemplate such factors as extensor mechanism management, exposure, implant removal and subsequent bone loss,

Dr. Newman or an immediate family member has received research or institutional support from Zimmer and Genzyme. Dr. Bezwada or an immediate family member is a member of a speakers' bureau or has made paid presentations on behalf of Genzyme, Sanofi-Aventis, and Biomet.

FIGURE 1

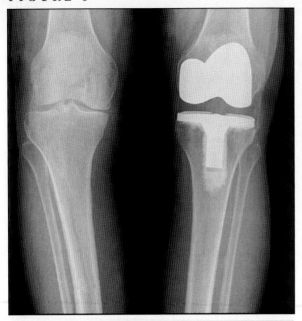

AP radiograph of the knees of a 67-year-old man who had continued global pain 4 years after total knee arthroplasty. Sometimes determining the reason for failure is not straightforward. Although the knee appears satisfactory on this radiograph, exhaustive history and physical examination revealed flexion instability.

FIGURE 2

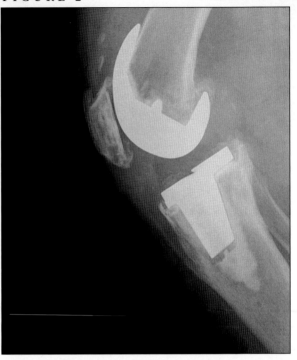

Lateral radiograph of the knee of a 74-year-old woman 12 years after total knee arthroplasty demonstrates obvious loosening of both the femoral and tibial stems with subsidence of bone overgrowth. Before diagnosis of aseptic loosening, infection should be ruled out.

component selection, reestablishing the joint line, and gap balancing for any underlying ligamentous deficiency. Anticipating all possibilities and having all necessary equipment on hand, including implant removal tools and implant options, will enhance the probability of a successful outcome.

UNDERSTANDING REASONS FOR FAILURE
History

The first step in determining the reasons for failure of a TKA is obtaining a complete history. Elements to include are chief symptom (pain, lack of motion, instability); number of prior operations; prior infections with any accompanying fevers, nausea, vomiting, or chills at the time of presentation; and the date of the last surgery. Further questioning for signs of infection should be sought, such as prior wound complications, prolonged wound drainage, or prolonged antibiotic treatment (**Figure 3**). The nature and duration of symptoms can also give clues to the underlying reason for failure. The timing of pain is essential; for instance, is the pain constant, or is it start-up pain? Is the pain isolated, or is it global? Is there associated swelling? Does the patient have giving-way symptoms? If so, in what position does this usually occur? It is also helpful to complete a nutritional assessment as well as a neurologic and peripheral vascular evaluation to uncover conditions that could portend poorer outcomes. Interest in possible metal sensitivity has increased recently with the newer components, especially metal-on-metal hip designs.[5] Questions should be asked about prior symptoms of metal allergy; further testing is appropriate if allergy is suspected. Simple questions can often help determine the likelihood of definitive diagnosis of failure and direct the workup going forward.

FIGURE 3

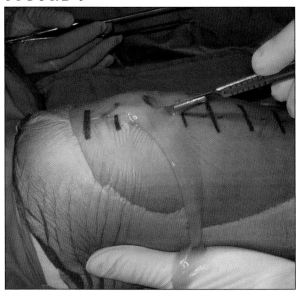

Photograph of an obviously infected TKA. When an infection is not this obvious, prior aspiration and blood work can help determine the diagnosis.

Physical Examination

The physical examination should begin with inspection, taking note of all previous incisions about the knee. The examiner should also inspect for any redness, swelling, drainage, or obvious deformity. Range of motion should be assessed, taking note of the stability of the knee in mid-flexion and at full flexion and extension. Standing alignment should be tested, which can give clues to ligamentous instability or component malalignment (**Figure 4**). Patellar maltracking or evidence of patellar clunk syndrome should be sought. The extensor mechanism should be tested to confirm that it is intact and functioning (**Figure 5**). Gait examination is very important; it can provide subtle clues to instability or malalignment of the implant. Special attention should be paid to a complete neurologic, motor, and peripheral vascular examination; problems in these areas could alter surgical outcomes. Surgeons should also seek other possible causes of referred pain; examination of the ipsilateral hip and spine is essential.

Laboratory Tests

Aspiration is warranted when a patient presents with almost any new symptom following a TKA. The fluid

FIGURE 4

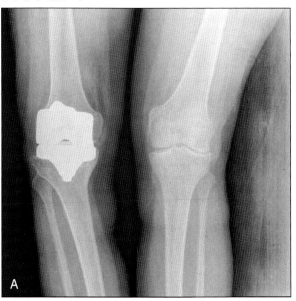
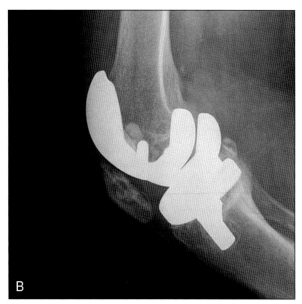

Radiographs of the knee of a 71-year-old woman who had continued deformity and pain with instability after total knee arthroplasty. **A**, AP radiograph reveals lateral laxity with malposition of the tibial component in varus alignment. **B**, Lateral radiograph illustrates varus tibial alignment and external rotation of the femoral component.

FIGURE 5

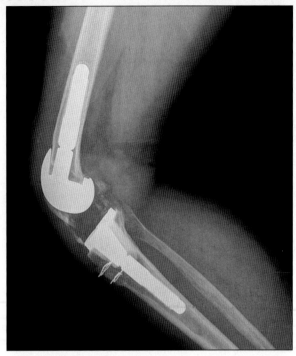

Lateral radiograph of the knee of a 57-year-old patient with extensor mechanism failure after previous revision TKA.

analysis can give clues to infection, and Gram stain, cell count, and aerobic and anaerobic cultures should be ordered. Schinsky et al[6] evaluated aspirations for suspected infection after total hip arthroplasty and found that synovial fluid cell counts of more than 3,000 white blood cells per milliliter combined with elevated CRP level and ESR was diagnostic of infection. In 2008, Ghanem et al[7] further evaluated the cell counts of suspected infection in TKAs. They found that fluid leukocyte counts greater than 1,100 cells/mL combined with neutrophil differential greater than 64% produced a 98.6% positive predictive value to diagnosing periprosthetic infection. These numbers, combined with simple blood tests such as an ESR and CRP level, can assist the surgeon in determining whether there is progression or resolution of symptoms and whether there is an infectious etiology. Increased attention is being paid to possible metal sensitivity testing, either serum or tissue sampling. Although it appears that patients with poor outcomes after TKA can have significant perivascular lymphocyte infiltration surrounding implants secondary to metal ions, it has not been determined if this represents a true metal allergy.[5]

Serial Radiographs

Serial radiographs can provide important clues with respect to a failed TKA. Mandatory radiographs include AP, lateral, and axial patellofemoral views. One can also consider long leg alignment films to determine any potential deformities. Plain radiographs can reveal osteolysis about the tibial or femoral component, polyethylene wear, rotational deformities, and patellar malalignment. The surgeon should also attempt to identify the components used, either with radiographic identification or from prior surgical reports. Knowing the track record of a particular component, the modes of failure associated with the device, and any nuances with regard to the modularity of the implant can be quite helpful.[8] Dynamic fluoroscopy or stress radiographs can be beneficial to determine instability of the implant either in extension or flexion. Perfectly tangential views of the cement-bone interface can be useful to determine subtle osteolysis. Although rarely indicated, bone scan can also be useful to evaluate for loosening or search for occult infection. New modalities such as CT and MRI with metal suppression have been useful to determine malrotation, osteolysis, and metal staining or muscle necrosis indicative of possible metal sensitivity.

TREATMENT OPTIONS

After the clinician has performed a complete history and physical examination, obtained appropriate images, ordered the indicated laboratory tests, and defined the reason for failure, the most appropriate route of treatment can be determined. Nonsurgical treatment of a failed TKA is sometimes indicated in elderly patients, those with considerable comorbidities, or in patients with persistent complex regional pain syndrome. Antibiotic suppression in these individuals can sometimes be successful and avoid the physiologic stress of multiple procedures. If no underlying cause can be determined initially, nonsurgical treatment may also be warranted because poor results are obtained when revision surgery is performed solely for pain.[4]

Once the decision for revision has been made, the surgeon must determine the most appropriate surgical pro-

FIGURE 6

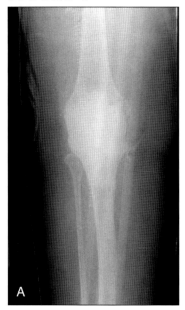

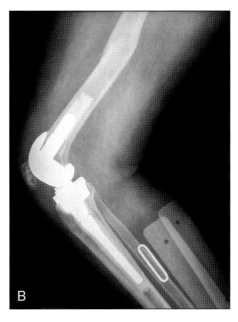

Radiographs of the knee of the patient shown in Figure 3, which was treated in a staged procedure. **A**, AP view shows the knee with a static spacer block in place. Note the large amount of bone loss that will need to be accommodated for during revision surgery. **B**, Lateral radiograph obtained after revision from static spacer. Bone loss necessitated the use of metal augments and long-stemmed implants.

cedure. Sometimes, clear polyethylene wear with no evidence of tibial or femoral loosening or malalignment can be treated successfully with simple polyethylene exchange with bone grafting of any obvious osteolysis. Engh et al,[8] however, found a significantly higher revision rate after simple polyethylene exchange in patients with accelerated wear, and they cautioned against this approach. If loosening or improper rotation of implants is obvious, however, then one- or two-stage revision is more appropriate. If there is any concern for infection, then two-stage revision with insertion of an articulating or static antibiotic cement spacer and intravenous antibiotic treatment until resolution is the most likely to yield good results (**Figure 6**). In the event of extensive bone loss in the setting of infection, a static spacer with intercalary nailing is a better option to prevent dislocation. One-stage revision can be quite successful if appropriate implants are selected and the clinician is able to obtain good soft-tissue balance and good motion and can appropriately address any bony defects in one surgical procedure.

PREOPERATIVE PLANNING

Preoperative planning is essential; the incision, exposure, prosthesis removal technique, bone defect reconstruc-

tion, and implant selection must be considered. The surgeon must remember to prepare for the worst and hope for the best. In facilities where many revisions are performed, the surgeon generally has access to several options for implants, bone grafting materials, and instruments to aid in implant removal. In lower-volume settings, however, preoperative planning and consultation with all appropriate company representatives to ensure access to needed instruments and implants can help avoid any delays or complications. It is generally advisable to perform appropriate planning at least 1 to 2 weeks before surgery and to augment this with radiographic rounds or multidisciplinary rounds that involve the entire surgical team (nurses, physical therapists, vendors) to help facilitate not only the surgical procedure but also the postoperative care of the patient.

REVISION SURGERY

Patient positioning for revision TKA is similar to that for primary TKA. The position should allow the surgeon to place the knee in the most appropriate position with the knee in hyperflexion. This can be facilitated with the use of a foot support to help hold the knee at 90°, or the use of additional surgical assistants. A tourniquet is

FIGURE 7

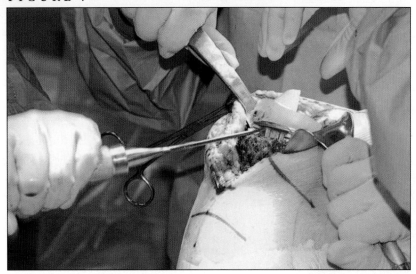

Intraoperative photograph demonstrates implant removal. Note that the cement–base plate interval needs to be broken before attempted implant removal to avoid bone loss.

advised in all but the rarest occasions, such as prior arterial repair or several peripheral vascular diseases with extensive calcification. Proper padding of all bony prominences is appropriate, as surgical times can be long and skin breakdown of normal skin is a risk.

Many patients who have had TKA have a history of multiple surgical procedures on the knee and thus have several incisions about the anterior aspect of the knee. A critical step in performing a successful revision is selecting the most appropriate incision to use. The most significant blood supply to the knee comes from the medial side and thus it may be most appropriate to use the most laterally based incision to allow for skin healing. If this is not possible, then leaving a skin bridge of at least 8 cm will decrease the risk of skin slough or wound breakdown. Also, any noted transverse incisions should be crossed at right angles, again to avoid any postoperative skin problems. In some patients with multiple prior incisions, a sham incision can be performed several weeks before the planned revision, to evaluate the potential for healing. In the setting of severely compromised skin or with prior infection and chronic wounds, it is advisable to consult a plastic surgeon either preoperatively or at the time of revision for possible flap coverage or the use of soft-tissue expanders. In general, small incisions should be avoided in revision surgery; it is best to extend the incision up to 5 cm both proximally

and distally to allow for proper removal and reinsertion of implants and to allow definition of proper tissue planes. The surgeon should be well versed in gaining exposure and should have a protocol that includes using a maximal incision into the extensor mechanism to mobilize both proximally and distally, elevating the fat pad and patellar tendon (often protecting this with a bone clamp or pin) and reestablishing the medial and lateral gutters. One can also consider performing a quadriceps snip with almost no extensor compromise; however, patellar turndown can often lead to postoperative extensor lag of 10° or more. Patellar eversion is not necessary in every procedure, as subluxation can suffice and can be facilitated with an inside-out lateral release. Occasionally, a tibial tubercle osteotomy or quadriceps turndown is needed to gain appropriate exposure. Some authors advocate a combined approach, elevating the extensor insertion along with the periosteum (the "banana peel" exposure), although with proper technique this is rarely required.

Implant removal is often tedious and can be fraught with complications. The goal of implant removal should be avoidance or minimization of host bone loss. In the setting of cemented implants, it is advisable to first attempt to break the implant-cement interface rather than the cement-bone interface, which can significantly damage the underlying bone (**Figure 7**). Again, the most appropriate first step in implant removal is adequate exposure. If greater exposure is needed, then a larger incision or mobilization of scar tissue is imperative. Several instruments can assist in this step. Micro oscillating saws, flexible chisels, and osteotomes are generally adequate to accomplish implant removal. Gigli saws should be avoided because they can remove excessive bone. Rigid extractors should never be used before breaking all points of fixation in the implant.

FIGURE 8

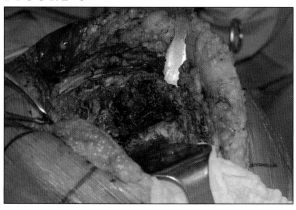

Intraoperative photograph illustrates the extensive bone loss after femoral implant removal. Note that bony landmarks for referencing have been obliterated; intramedullary referencing is requisite.

Host bone loss and prior arthroplasty can often obscure the standard referencing points (**Figure 8**), making the use of posterior or anterior referencing or the Whiteside line difficult. The epicondylar axis may be intact; however, because long-stemmed revision implants are generally used, intramedullary referencing instruments are usually more accurate (**Figure 9**). The goal after removal should be to balance both the flexion and extension gap, and it is appropriate to first address the tibia and create a platform for femoral reconstruction.

Once appropriate removal of implants and re-creation of the flexion and extension gaps has been performed, the next critical step is to address any bony defects. The surgeon must keep in mind that during bone defect augmentation, re-creation of the joint line can influence both the flexion and extension balancing (**Figure 10**). Because of this, our approach is to determine the flexion gap first. This facilitates extension balancing because it decreases the number of variables available to change—distal femoral cuts, distal femoral augments, and polyethylene thickness. If the knee is stable in both flexion and extension at this point, then implant insertion can proceed. If the flexion gap is adequate and it is loose in extension, then adding distal augments is appropriate. Last, if flexion is adequate but the knee is tight in extension, then additional distal resection is needed.

FIGURE 9

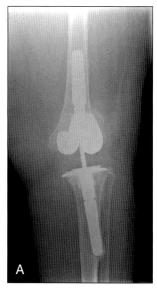
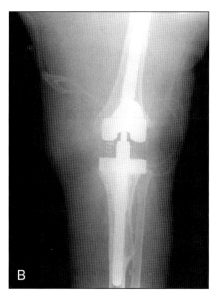

AP radiographs of a knee in which revision TKA failed. **A**, Note obvious tibial component loosening. During surgery, all bony landmarks were altered; intramedullary referencing and long-stemmed components are needed. **B**, After revision using tibial metal buildup, thick polyethylene, and long-stemmed components bypassing the area of obvious loosening.

FIGURE 10

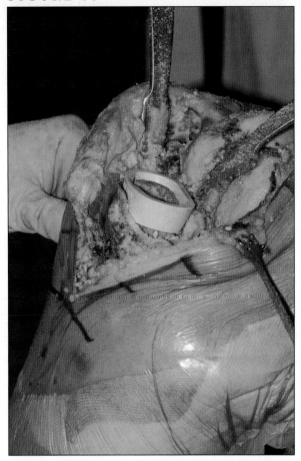

Intraoperative photograph shows placement of metal augment on the tibia, re-creating the joint line and allowing gap balancing to commence.

Several options for addressing bony defects or gap imbalance are available, including metal augments, allograft, or cement. Most contemporary revision systems allow metal augments to be screwed onto the revision components, and these systems provide cutting guides to appropriately prepare the host bone. With cavitary bone defects, impaction grafting can be performed with cancellous bone, followed by cementing of the prosthesis onto and into the impacted bone. Because this technique is often difficult and can lead to iatrogenic fractures, caution is advised. With severe bone loss, structural allografts with a constrained device can be used. This requires special expertise, however, and generally should be considered only by an experienced revision knee arthroplasty surgeon. The last option is distal femoral replacement, but this is generally considered a salvage procedure, and special equipment and implants are needed.

After appropriate implant removal and augmentation of bone defects, implant selection is the next step. Long-stemmed press-fit devices are the most appropriate, along with cement augmentation of the tibial and femoral baseplate. Posterior cruciate–substituting devices are used almost exclusively and help facilitate soft-tissue balancing. In cases of severe soft-tissue laxity or severe bone loss, either a constrained condylar device or hinged device can be used; however, this is at the expense of losing knee kinematics. The patellar component is usually the last to be addressed. The first step should be to determine the patellar component thickness; bone surface should be a minimum of 10 mm. Revision knee arthroplasty outcomes are better when the patella is resurfaced, in terms of both reducing anterior knee pain and restoring alignment and mechanics of the extensor mechanism. However, Lonner et al[9] have shown that the retention of a well-positioned, stable all-polyethylene patellar component can be successful and that revision is not always necessary. If revision of the patellar component is needed, however, care must be taken to avoid excessive resection of patellar bone stock and thus avoid osteonecrosis.

POSTOPERATIVE CARE

In general, the postoperative protocol for revision surgery is similar to that for primary surgery. The patient may begin to bear weight immediately, unless a tibial tubercle osteotomy was performed or extensive allograft was used, which may necessitate toe-touch weight bearing for 6 to 8 weeks and the use of a knee immobilizer. Continuous passive motion devices can be used, but again care must be taken if allograft was used or an osteotomy or quadriceps snip was performed. Parenteral antibiotics are usually continued for 3 to 5 days, or until intraoperative cultures are final. Deep vein thrombosis prophylaxis is also recommended, but use of low-molecular-weight heparin, warfarin, or compression devices is debatable, as is duration of treatment. Skin staples or sutures are generally removed at 2 weeks, and early follow-up at 4 to 6 weeks and again at 3 months is advisable.

CLINICAL RESULTS

Primary TKA has an unparalleled track record for function and pain relief, approaching 95% good and excellent long-term results; however, revision TKA has only 81% good and excellent long-term results.[10] Failed primary TKA requiring revision is associated with multiple factors, including bone loss, ligament balance, soft-tissue coverage, patellofemoral articulation, and integrity of the extensor mechanism. Also, patients who undergo revision are generally elderly and have more underlying comorbid conditions, and the increased surgical time and complexity lead to poorer long-term outcomes. When an etiology for failure can be identified, however, outcomes improve. Revisions for arthrofibrosis show significant improvements in the mean Knee Society pain score as well as overall arc of motion, leading to modest improvements.[11] However, Mont et al[4] reported that patients who underwent revision for pain and stiffness gained only about 40° of motion and only 60% were considered to have good or excellent outcomes. In addition, patients who underwent revision only for unexplained pain fared far worse.[4] In contrast, patients identified as having mechanical failure, instability, or wear and loosening had the best outcomes with respect to postoperative pain and functional scores. Schwab et al[12] reported on 10 patients who underwent revision surgery for instability. Pain scores improved significantly, along with stability, and 9 of 10 patients reported satisfaction. Mabry et al[13] reported the results in 73 knees in 72 patients. Three patients died or were followed less than 2 years; the other 70 knees in 69 patients had a median follow-up of 10.2 years. Four knees underwent both femoral and tibial rerevisions for recurrent aseptic loosening, and one patella was rerevised for loosening and polyethylene wear, for a 92% survivorship at 10 years. Haas et al[14] reported 56 (84%) good or excellent results in 67 knees revised for aseptic loosening with cemented modular components.

Infection after total joint arthroplasty is a devastating problem. The goals of surgery in the infected knee change from pain relief and function to obtaining a knee replacement free of infection. Meek et al[15] reported that functional outcome in 47 patients treated with two-stage revision improved range of motion modestly (from 78 to 87 at 2 years), and pain scores were improved. Good results can be obtained for nearly all revision TKAs with proper use of the following principles: identification of the etiology for failure, proper preoperative planning, and meticulous surgical technique. With the number of revisions likely to increase dramatically, it behooves the revision surgeon to be well versed in these principles and be able to apply them properly.

REFERENCES

1. Kurtz S, Mowat F, Ong K, Chan N, Lau E, Halpern M: Prevalence of primary and revision total hip and knee arthroplasty in the United States from 1990 through 2002. *J Bone Joint Surg Am* 2005;87(7):1487-1497.

2. Kurtz S, Ong K, Lau E, Mowat F, Halpern M: Projections of primary and revision hip and knee arthroplasty in the United States from 2005 to 2030. *J Bone Joint Surg Am* 2007;89(4):780-785.

3. Gonzalez MH, Mekhail AO: The failed total knee arthroplasty: Evaluation and etiology. *J Am Acad Orthop Surg* 2004;12(6):436-446.

4. Mont MA, Serna FK, Krackow KA, Hungerford DS: Exploration of radiographically normal total knee replacements for unexplained pain. *Clin Orthop Relat Res* 1996;331(331):216-220.

5. Hallab NJ, Caicedo M, Finnegan A, Jacobs JJ: Th1 type lymphocyte reactivity to metals in patients with total hip arthroplasty. *J Orthop Surg Res* 2008;3:6.

6. Schinsky MF, Della Valle CJ, Sporer SM, Paprosky WG: Perioperative testing for joint infection in patients undergoing revision total hip arthroplasty. *J Bone Joint Surg Am* 2008;90(9):1869-1875.

7. Ghanem E, Parvizi J, Burnett RS, et al: Cell count and differential of aspirated fluid in the diagnosis of infection at the site of total knee arthroplasty. *J Bone Joint Surg Am* 2008;90(8):1637-1643.

8. Engh GA, Koralewicz LM, Pereles TR: Clinical results of modular polyethylene insert exchange with retention of total knee arthroplasty components. *J Bone Joint Surg Am* 2000;82(4):516-523.

9. Lonner JH, Mont MA, Sharkey PF, Siliski JM, Rajadhyaksha AD, Lotke PA: Fate of the unrevised all-polyethylene patellar component in revision total knee arthroplasty. *J Bone Joint Surg Am* 2003;85-A(1):56-59.

10. Hanssen AD, Rand JA: A comparison of primary and revision total knee arthroplasty using the kinematic stabilizer prosthesis. *J Bone Joint Surg Am* 1988;70(4):491-499.

11. Kim J, Nelson CL, Lotke PA: Stiffness after total knee arthroplasty: Prevalence of the complication and outcomes of revision. *J Bone Joint Surg Am* 2004;86-A(7): 1479-1484.

12. Schwab JH, Haidukewych GJ, Hanssen AD, Jacofsky DJ, Pagnano MW: Flexion instability without dislocation after posterior stabilized total knees. *Clin Orthop Relat Res* 2005;440:96-100.

13. Mabry TM, Vessely MB, Schleck CD, Harmsen WS, Berry DJ: Revision total knee arthroplasty with modular cemented stems: Long-term follow-up. *J Arthroplasty* 2007;22(6, Suppl 2)100-105.

14. Haas SB, Insall JN, Montgomery W III, Windsor RE: Revision total knee arthroplasty with use of modular components with stems inserted without cement. *J Bone Joint Surg Am* 1995;77(11):1700-1707.

15. Meek RM, Masri BA, Dunlop D, et al: Patient satisfaction and functional status after treatment of infection at the site of a total knee arthroplasty with use of the PROSTALAC articulating spacer. *J Bone Joint Surg Am* 2003;85-A(10):1888-1892.

CHAPTER 2

PREOPERATIVE PLANNING FOR REVISION TOTAL KNEE ARTHROPLASTY

WADIH Y. MATAR, MD, MSC, FRCSC

INTRODUCTION

The number of revision total knee arthroplasties (TKAs) performed is expected to increase drastically over the next few decades.[1,2] Therefore, as the revision surgeon's workload grows, it becomes increasingly important to perform revision TKA in an efficient manner while minimizing the risks and potential complications. Developing a thorough and precise surgical plan preoperatively helps achieve these goals, contributing to a good outcome following the revision surgery.

The preoperative process, as outlined in this chapter, begins with a detailed history and physical examination. These are complemented by an analysis of laboratory results and radiologic findings to ascertain the proper indication for the revision surgery. Finally, a plan is developed with the surgical team. This plan should address ordering the proper extraction equipment for the implant in situ, as well as the instruments, implants, and grafts needed for the revision surgery.

HISTORY

History taking revolves around asking questions about the presenting symptoms to better understand the cause of the TKA failure. Indications for TKA revisions are numerous; leading causes include infection, malalignment, malpositioning, instability, periprosthetic fracture, stiffness, and aseptic loosening.[3] Revisions for unexplained pain are rarely successful; hence, it is important to establish the correct diagnosis. The decision to proceed with revision TKA is made in concert with the patient and is subject to the same contraindications as a primary TKA, such as a vascularly compromised limb, certain infections, Charcot arthropathy, and some neuromuscular diseases.[4] Special attention should also be paid to the patient's general medical condition and nutritional status. If these cannot be corrected, the patient should not be offered revision surgery, as several studies have shown the negative effects of malnutrition following total joint arthroplasty.[5-7]

Questions about the onset, duration, pattern, and intensity of the symptoms should be asked, as well as questions about alleviating and provoking factors. The timing of the onset of the symptoms is especially important, as ongoing symptoms since the primary TKA are suggestive of infection or extra-articularly referred causes, whereas symptoms appearing years after a symptom-free period may be suggestive of sepsis by hematogenous seeding or osteolysis causing instability and component loosening. Symptoms of knee buckling or giving way are consistent with TKA instability. Constitutional symptoms, such as fever or chills, are red flags for TKA sepsis. Questions should also be directed toward the hip and lower back to rule out pain radiating to the knee. Last, the effect that the symptoms have

---

Neither Dr. Matar nor any immediate family member has received anything of value from or owns stock in a commercial company or institution related directly or indirectly to the subject of this chapter.

on the patient's lifestyle, activities of daily living, and mobility also should be questioned.

The surgeon should review previous clinical notes and surgical reports to identify any preexisting clinical issues or any complications, such as soft-tissue disruption, encountered during the index procedure. Previous surgical reports are also examined to find out the specific implant manufacturer, type, and size. The surgeon needs to be familiar with the implants in situ with regard to their availability, modularity, and polyethylene locking mechanism, and their most common modes of failure. If the surgeon decides to perform a partial revision (eg, polyethylene liner exchange), the specific replacement implants need to be ordered before the procedure. In some cases, the replacement implants will no longer be available, forcing the surgeon to perform a full revision.

Physical Examination

Physical examination begins with an overall assessment of the patient, including height and weight. Special attention is then given to the lower limb, especially the overall leg alignment, with the patient in the standing and supine positions. The active and passive range of motion of the knee is measured with the aid of a goniometer. Special consideration is given to stiffness, which may require a more extensile exposure and possibly some ligamentous and capsular releases. An extensor lag may represent a compromised extensor mechanism. Knee stability is checked in the coronal and sagittal planes. Coronal plane stability (varus/valgus) is checked with the knee in full extension and in 30° of flexion. Instability, if present, should be quantified in degrees and evaluated for the presence of a soft or hard end point. Coronal plane instability may need to be addressed by implanting a more constrained device. Sagittal plane stability (anterior/posterior) is checked with the knee in full extension as well as 30° and 90° of flexion. Measurement of instability is quite subjective, so stability should be reassessed intraoperatively. Instability should be addressed during the revision surgery by carefully balancing the flexion and extension gaps or by implanting a more constrained device, such as a posteriorly stabilized device, in a posterior cruciate ligament–deficient cruciate-retaining TKA. Patellar tracking is also evaluated by actively and passively cycling the patient's knee. Maltracking, if present, should be investigated for possible causes such as femoral implant malrotation and should be corrected during the revision surgery.

The knee's soft-tissue status and adhesions to underlying structures also are examined, and all previous surgical scars are inspected (**Figure 1**). When faced with multiple incisions, the surgeon should use the most lateral and anterior scar to diminish the potential for wound necrosis and maximize healing. When in doubt, the surgeon might consider a sham incision or a preoperative evaluation by a plastic surgeon for consideration of a gastrocnemius flap or use of a soft-tissue expander before proceeding with the planned revision TKA. In complicated infection cases with extensor mechanism compromise, where reconstruction may not be feasible, the arthroplasty surgeon, after consultation with a plastic surgeon, might opt for lifelong suppressive antibiotics or consider a fusion or an above-knee amputation.

An overall assessment of the hip and spine is performed to rule out referred pathology. Last, the neurovascular status of the lower limb is evaluated. Any neurologic findings should prompt further investigations (eg, electromyography or spine MRI) and an evaluation by a neurologist for a possible neurologic disorder. An absent or diminished dorsalis pedis or posterior tibialis pulse or changes consistent with peripheral vascular disease warrant a preoperative vascular evaluation beginning with noninvasive testing, possibly followed by a lower limb arteriogram.

Imaging Studies

The standard weight-bearing AP, lateral, and patellofemoral (skyline) radiographic views are essential (**Figure 2**). The quality and technique of the radiographs should be adequate, and the radiographs should show normal diaphysis above the femoral implant and below the tibial prosthesis. The radiographs are assessed for overall mechanical coronal limb alignment. If needed, 36-in (full-length) weight-bearing AP radiographs also can be obtained. The latter view is also examined for the angle of the distal femoral resection as well as the presence of any femoral or tibial diaphyseal deformities. Other views, such as dynamic views in cases of instability, may be helpful in some situations. CT scans also can be useful when implant malrotation is suspected.

Radiographs are assessed for manufacturer, type, and size of the implant. When available, old surgical records or implant labels from the index procedure greatly facilitate this process. If these are not available and the specific implant cannot be identified by examining the radiographs, the surgeon should compare the radiographs with an implant atlas or show them to colleagues or manufacturers' representatives for identification. Following the identification of the implant, the radiographs are examined for the positioning and alignment of implants. The joint-line height is also assessed. The lateral radiograph is further examined for patellar height and sagittal component alignment. The skyline view is examined for patellar bone stock and patellar position over the femoral component, as well as the

FIGURE 1

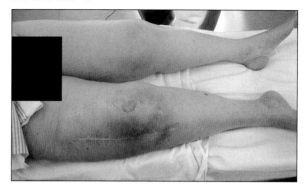

Photograph shows limb with previous surgical incisions before revision total knee arthroplasty.

FIGURE 2

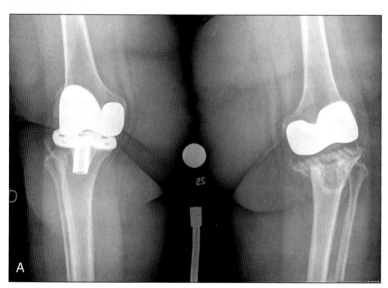

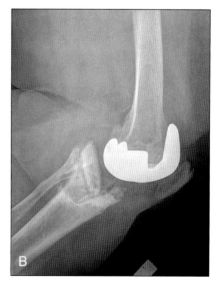

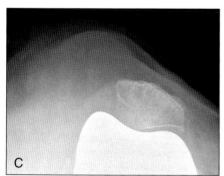

Radiographs obtained before revision TKA should include a weight-bearing AP view (**A**), a lateral view (**B**), and a patellofemoral (skyline) view (**C**). This series shows catastrophic failure of an all-polyethylene tibial component with loosening, metaphyseal bone loss, instability, and malalignment.

medial-lateral position of the patellar implant on the patella. Any discrepancies should be addressed during the revision surgery; however, the surgeon might opt to keep the same patellar implant despite revising both the tibial and femoral implants, if the position and fixation of the patellofemoral implant are adequate and the implant in situ is compatible with the revised femoral component.

Implant fixation and osteolysis leading to bone loss, implant loosening, and ultimate implant failure also should be carefully examined. Implant fixation is first assessed by looking at the cement-bone interface in a cemented TKA or the implant-bone interface in an uncemented TKA on the AP and lateral views. It is crucial to make sure that these radiographs are obtained with the x-ray beam parallel to the tibial base plate on the AP view and parallel to the femoral implant on the lateral view because an obliquely oriented beam will not adequately display the interface and may fail to show early signs of loosening (radiolucent lines). The surgeon should also examine historical radiographs for progression of radiolucent lines to document progression of implant migration in cases of loosening. Careful attention also should be paid to osteolytic lesions, as these can be obstructed by the implant or cement and therefore need to be better visualized using oblique radiographs[8] or with the help of CT scans using metal-suppression software. The size and location of the bone loss is identified, and this information is used to plan the grafts or augments needed during the revision surgery. The Anderson Orthopaedic Research Institute (AORI) bone defect classification system is used to document and better characterize the defects intraoperatively.[9]

To differentiate between aseptic loosening and prosthetic joint infection, nuclear medicine scans should be used with caution because of their suboptimal sensitivity and specificity and because the scans may remain positive for a prolonged period of time following the index procedure.[10,11] Bone scintigraphy has a high negative predictive value, making a negative scan a good indicator of the absence of major problems following TKA; however, its accuracy is low, at 50% to 70%. Combining the bone scan with gallium scan improves its accuracy only slightly, to 65% to 80%; therefore, these tests should be considered good screening tests for TKA pathologies.

LABORATORY ANALYSIS

All TKA revision patients should be evaluated preoperatively by an internal medicine or cardiology consultant for assessment and, if needed, optimization of health status before the surgery. The American College of Cardiology/American Heart Association (ACC/AHA) publishes perioperative cardiac assessment guidelines that can be used to evaluate the patient preoperatively and to make recommendations regarding the appropriate testing that is likely to best guide patient treatment.[12] These guidelines have been shown to accurately predict perioperative cardiac risk in the orthopaedic patient.[13] During the preoperative evaluation, routine testing (eg, blood work, electrocardiogram, chest radiographs) is done, with more invasive testing performed as needed according to the patient's comorbidities. Basic blood work includes a complete blood cell count with a differential, renal and hepatic function tests, blood chemistry, coagulation studies, and inflammatory markers. The latter, consisting of the erythrocyte sedimentation rate (ESR) and C-reactive protein (CRP) level, are used to screen for the presence of periprosthetic infection (PPI). Recently, Ghanem et al[14] showed that an ESR value greater than 30 mm/h had a sensitivity of 94.3% in diagnosing PPI, and a CRP value above 10 mg/L had a sensitivity of 91.1%, with the combination of both values increasing the sensitivity to detect infection to 97.6%. When faced with ESR and/or CRP values above these thresholds, or when the diagnosis of infection is highly suspected, a knee aspiration is performed, because bacterial cultures remain the gold standard test for establishing the diagnosis of PPI. The aspirate should also be sent for leukocyte cell count and differential, given that at times the cultures do not grow bacteria, such as in cases of prior antibiotic exposure. Using receiver operating characteristic curves, Ghanem et al[15] calculated that a cell count of $1,100$ cells/$10,000$ mL^3 or greater and a neutrophil differential 64% or greater were accurate in diagnosing PPI, with a positive predictive value of 98.6% when both values were above their cutoffs.

The patient's nutritional status also should be assessed. If the serum transferrin level is less than 200 mg/dL, serum albumin is below 3.5 g/dL, or total lymphocyte count is less than 1,500/mm^3, the diagnosis of malnutrition is considered and the patient should be assessed and treated by a nutritionist preoperatively.

REVISION TKA

Prior to proceeding with the revision surgery, the team should formulate a precise primary revision plan along with preparing some contingency plans if needed. For example, the anesthesia and postoperative care plans also should be discussed and formulated in cases in which an intensive care unit bed is likely to be required postoperatively. The preoperative planning is best performed in a case discussion manner with all members of the team present (surgeon, fellow, resident, surgical assistant, head nurse, operating room orthopaedic coordinator). The team should indicate the type and size of the implant in situ on the radiographs and template the radiographs with the proposed revision implants. These templates, along with detailed surgical plans that include the equipment and grafts needed, are then conveyed to the operating room staff and the implant manufacturer representatives to ensure that the proper equipment is available on the day of surgery.

On the morning of surgery, the surgeon should briefly review the history, physical examination, and laboratory findings along with the templated radiographs. The surgeon should also review the surgical plan with the anesthetist to determine the proper type and duration of the required anesthesia, along with the need for transfusion and cell-saver use if excessive blood loss is expected. The surgical team should also make sure that all ordered equipment and grafts are available before the induction of anesthesia. It is essential that surgery be delayed until all equipment is present and verified in the operating room, to prevent the catastrophic intraoperative situation in which the proper equipment or implants are not available.

Basic revision equipment is needed. This includes but is not limited to osteotomes, various saws (Gigli and power saws), burrs, metal-cutting disks, punches, and ultrasonic tools for cement removal. If an extraction tray specific to the implant in situ exists, it should be available in addition to the usual equipment needed for implant removal. When revising the femoral or tibial component, the chosen TKA revision system is usually modular and includes stems for diaphyseal fixation along with metal augments and metaphyseal sleeves in cases of metaphyseal bone loss. With a case of instability, massive bone loss, or ligamentous compromise, implants with increasing degrees of restraint, including

a hinged device, should be available for the operating surgeon. The implant company's representative should also be available during the surgery, especially if the operating room staff or nurses are not familiar with the equipment and implants.

CONCLUSIONS

By means of a detailed history, thorough physical examination, and appropriate testing, the arthroplasty surgeon should always establish the proper diagnosis before embarking on the revision surgery. Revision TKA surgery can often be complicated; however, its success and ease can be greatly enhanced by a well-formulated and precise preoperative plan. A highly trained operating room team in a high-volume center can greatly facilitate this process.

REFERENCES

1. Kurtz S, Ong K, Lau E, Mowat F, Halpern M: Projections of primary and revision hip and knee arthroplasty in the United States from 2005 to 2030. *J Bone Joint Surg Am* 2007;89(4):780-785.

2. Kurtz SM, Ong KL, Schmier J, et al: Future clinical and economic impact of revision total hip and knee arthroplasty. *J Bone Joint Surg Am* 2007;89(Suppl 3):144-151.

3. Sharkey PF, Hozack WJ, Rothman RH, Shastri S, Jacoby SM: Insall Award paper: Why are total knee arthroplasties failing today? *Clin Orthop Relat Res* 2002;404:7-13.

4. Dennis DA, Berry DJ, Engh G, et al: Revision total knee arthroplasty. *J Am Acad Orthop Surg* 2008;16(8): 442-454.

5. Lavernia CJ, Sierra RJ, Baerga L: Nutritional parameters and short term outcome in arthroplasty. *J Am Coll Nutr* 1999;18(3):274-278.

6. Greene KA, Wilde AH, Stulberg BN: Preoperative nutritional status of total joint patients: Relationship to postoperative wound complications. *J Arthroplasty* 1991;6(4):321-325.

7. Gherini S, Vaughn BK, Lombardi AV Jr, Mallory TH: Delayed wound healing and nutritional deficiencies after total hip arthroplasty. *Clin Orthop Relat Res* 1993;293:188-195.

8. Nadaud MC, Fehring TK, Fehring K: Underestimation of osteolysis in posterior stabilized total knee arthroplasty. *J Arthroplasty* 2004;19(1):110-115.

9. Engh GA: Bone defect classification, in Engh GA, Rorabeck CH, eds: *Revision in Total Knee Arthroplasty.* Baltimore, MD, Lippincott Williams & Wilkins, 1997, pp 63-120.

10. Rand JA, Brown ML: The value of indium 111 leukocyte scanning in the evaluation of painful or infected total knee arthroplasties. *Clin Orthop Relat Res* 1990;259:179-182.

11. Love C, Marwin SE, Palestro CJ: Nuclear medicine and the infected joint replacement. *Semin Nucl Med* 2009;39(1):66-78.

12. Fleisher LA, Beckman JA, Brown KA, et al: ACC/AHA 2007 guidelines on perioperative cardiovascular evaluation and care for noncardiac surgery: A report of the American College of Cardiology/American Heart Association Task Force on Practice Guidelines (Writing Committee to Revise the 2002 Guidelines on Perioperative Cardiovascular Evaluation for Noncardiac Surgery). *Circulation* 2007;116(17):e418-e499.

13. Salerno SM, Carlson DW, Soh EK, Lettieri CJ: Impact of perioperative cardiac assessment guidelines on management of orthopedic surgery patients. *Am J Med* 2007;120(2):185-186, e1-e6.

14. Ghanem E, Antoci V Jr, Pulido L, Joshi A, Hozack W, Parvizi J: The use of receiver operating characteristics analysis in determining erythrocyte sedimentation rate and C-reactive protein levels in diagnosing periprosthetic infection prior to revision total hip arthroplasty. *Int J Infect Dis* 2009;13(6):e444-e449.

15. Ghanem E, Parvizi J, Burnett RS, et al: Cell count and differential of aspirated fluid in the diagnosis of infection at the site of total knee arthroplasty. *J Bone Joint Surg Am* 2008;90(8):1637-1643.

CHAPTER *3*

EXPOSURE FOR REVISION TOTAL KNEE ARTHROPLASTY

CRAIG J. DELLA VALLE, MD

INTRODUCTION

Adequate exposure and proper visualization are critical in revision total knee arthroplasty (TKA). The primary goals of exposure are to visualize the components that are presently in place so that they can be removed safely (without damage to the remaining host bone stock) and to allow for accurate implantation of the revision components. The surgeon must avoid damage to the skin and the extensor mechanism during this process, as injury to either of these structures can lead to complications (infection and extensor mechanism disruption, respectively) that are among the most challenging to manage. Further, these two complications can irrevocably change the prognosis for the patient's final outcome.

The exposure should be chosen as part of the preoperative plan, which typically should include a stepwise strategy for how exposure will be managed if difficulties are encountered. In patients with immobile and/or indurated skin around the prior incision, with multiple prior incisions, or with an active or healed sinus, serious consideration should be given to preoperative consultation with an orthopaedic hand surgeon or plastic surgeon who can assist with wound closure in the form of a muscle flap (typically, a medial gastrocnemius muscle flap[1-3]) or plan for a staged reconstruction with a skin expander[4-7] if necessary. In addition to the aforementioned risk factors for difficulties with exposure or

wound closure, patients with multiple prior surgeries, poor range of motion, heterotopic ossification, a history of radiation to the knee, or patella infera are likewise at increased risk for wound healing complications, and a difficult exposure should be anticipated (**Figure 1**).

SKIN INCISION

The first decision that the revision surgeon must make is where to make the skin incision. In patients with a single midline incision, the decision is straightforward; however, in patients with multiple prior incisions, the decision-making process can be more complex. In general, the surgeon should choose the most lateral incision available because the blood supply to the anterior aspect of the knee is derived medially and a more medial incision can lead to necrosis of the skin on the lateral side of the knee.[8,9] The age of the incision also should be considered. Older incisions (more than 20 years old) can be ignored more safely than more recent ones, for which inadequate time has elapsed for the subdermal plexus to revascularize areas where flaps have been raised (**Figure 2**).

If a second incision must be made, such as in a patient with a prior incision too far lateral to safely perform the revision procedure, a skin bridge of 6 to 8 cm is recommended. A prior transverse incision, such as from a previous high tibial osteotomy or patellectomy, can generally be crossed perpendicularly without causing

Dr. Della Valle or an immediate family member serves as a board member, owner, officer, or committee member of the American Association of Hip and Knee Surgeons and the Arthritis Foundation; serves as a paid consultant to or is an employee of Angiotech, Biomet, Kinamed, Smith & Nephew, and Zimmer; and has received research or institutional support from Pacira and Zimmer.

FIGURE 1

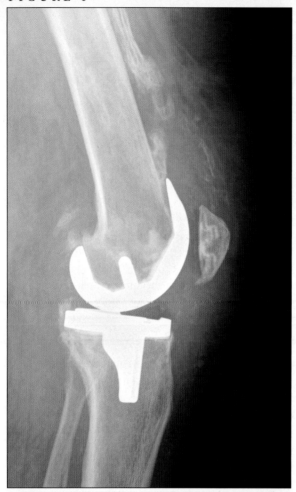

Lateral radiograph of the knee of a patient with stiffness shows severe heterotopic ossification. Difficulties with exposure should be anticipated.

FIGURE 2

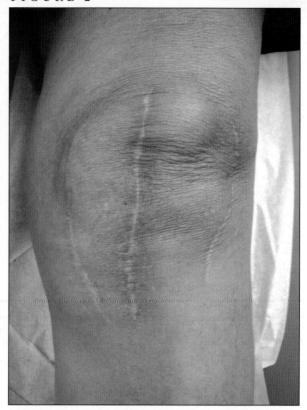

Photograph shows the knee of a patient with three prior skin incisions on the anterior aspect of the knee. The medial and lateral incisions were more than 20 years old. The central incision, which was 8 years old, was chosen for exposure.

wound healing problems.[10] Small oblique scars, such as from an open meniscectomy, can generally be ignored. If larger scars are encountered, however, the surgeon should avoid creating sharp angles (< ~60°), to decrease the risk of skin necrosis.

When making the skin incision, it is critical to create full-thickness skin flaps in continuity with the superficial fascia (**Figure 3**). The blood supply to the skin runs from the deeper tissues (it does not run superficially),

and thus subcutaneous flaps must be avoided. In general, skin flaps are raised only far enough to both make and easily close the arthrotomy, by exposing about 1 cm on either side of the proposed deep dissection.

MEDIAL PARAPATELLAR APPROACH

A medial parapatellar approach is the workhorse of revision TKA exposures and is adequate for the vast majority of revision procedures. Some surgeons may have expertise with the midvastus or subvastus approach to the knee, but the medial parapatellar approach, being the most extensile, is recommended for revision TKAs.

FIGURE 3

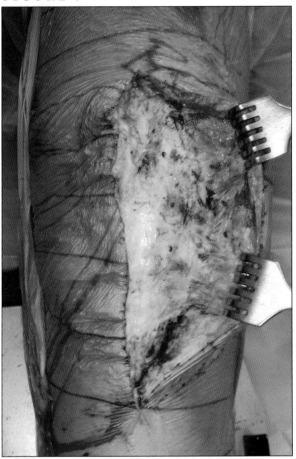

Intraoperative photograph shows full-thickness skin flaps.

Technique

The arthrotomy is made from the medial border of the apex of the quadriceps tendon, continues along the medial border of the patella, and ends along the medial aspect of the tibial tubercle (**Figure 4, *A***). Next, a subperiosteal dissection is performed along the medial aspect of the tibia (**Figure 4, *B***). A full-thickness release of the medial soft tissues from the proximal aspect of the tibia is performed, typically with electrocautery, and is completed with a curved osteotome around the posteromedial corner of the tibia to the semimembranosus insertion. The medial soft-tissue release is critical to eas-

ing exposure; it allows the surgeon to externally rotate the tibia, which will decrease tension on the extensor mechanism and improve visualization.

Following this release, a complete anterior synovectomy is performed, reestablishing the suprapatellar pouch and the medial and lateral gutters. The first step in this process is to identify the interval between the scar and the overlying medial capsular tissues on the medial side or the extensor mechanism on the lateral side of the arthrotomy (**Figure 4, *C***). The scar in this area is then resected (**Figure 4, *D***), which greatly improves both the mobility of the extensor mechanism and the exposure. Next, the surgeon can develop the plane underneath the extensor mechanism proximally, essentially performing a quadricepsplasty (**Figure 4, *E***). It is important, however, not to subperiosteally strip soft tissue from the anterior aspect of the femur itself, as this can lead to excessive bleeding and recurrent scar tissue in the suprapatellar pouch.

The interval behind the patellar tendon is then cleared by resecting additional scar tissue and releasing the soft tissue from the lateral side of the proximal tibia behind the patellar tendon; this greatly enhances exposure by mobilizing the patellar tendon (**Figure 4, *C*** and ***F***). Finally, the modular polyethylene liner is removed (**Figure 4, *G***). Before entering the operating room, the surgeon should know what kind of prosthesis is presently implanted so that a surgical plan is in place for how to defeat the polyethylene liner locking mechanism. At this point, an attempt is made to subluxate the patella laterally; in most cases, adequate exposure will have been obtained (**Figure 4, *H***). Although the patella can be everted, subluxation usually allows adequate exposure without placing excessive tension on the patellar tendon.

If at this point the patella will not subluxate or exposure is otherwise suboptimal, a lateral retinacular peel or formal lateral retinacular release can be performed. If a large amount of bone is present lateral to the implanted patellar component, it can be resected with an oscillating saw, taking care to not damage the polyethylene button. In most cases this is not required, however, as peeling soft tissue off the lateral border of the patella will increase patellar mobility enough that exposure can be obtained (**Figure 4, *I***). If exposure is still suboptimal, then a formal lateral retinacular release can be performed either from inside out (which is preferred)

FIGURE 4

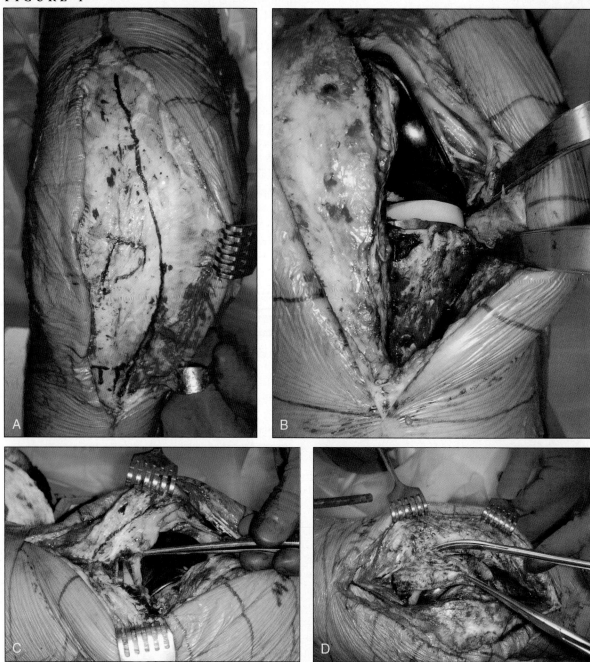

Intraoperative photographs show exposure for revision total knee arthroplasty through a medial parapatellar approach. **A**, The arthrotomy is performed along the medial border of the rectus femoris tendon, around the patella (marked P), and to the medial border of the tibial tubercle (marked TT). **B**, Medial subperiosteal dissection is performed. **C**, The interval between the patellar tendon and underlying scar is identified before removal. **D**, The scar underneath the medial aspect of the arthrotomy is resected.

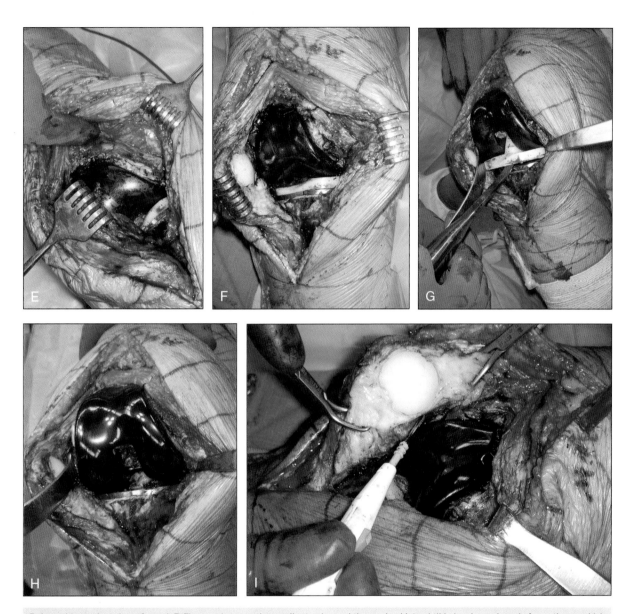

E, A quadricepsplasty is performed. **F**, The area between the patellar tendon and the proximal lateral tibia has been cleared of scar tissue, which vastly improves exposure. **G**, Removal of the modular polyethylene liner. **H**, The patella has been subluxated laterally, and adequate exposure has been obtained. **I**, Bone has been removed from the lateral border of the patella and associated scar tissue resected, which improves exposure.

or outside in. If an outside-in lateral retinacular release is performed, the surgeon should be aware that blood may pool underneath the skin, causing large areas of ecchymosis on the lateral aspect of the wound.[11]

Results

Sharkey et al[12] reported results at their institution using a medial parapatellar approach in conjunction with what they described as extensor mechanism tenolysis in a series of 207 consecutive revision TKAs. The approach described was adequate in 203 of these knees (98%); 2 knees required a V-Y quadricepsplasty turndown, and 2 required a patellectomy. In a similar report, Della Valle et al[13] described a single surgeon's experience with 126 consecutive revision TKAs. A medial capsular approach achieved adequate exposure in 111 of the 121 knees with an intact extensor mechanism. A quadriceps snip was required in 9 patients, and a lateral parapatellar approach was used in 1 patient because the primary TKA was done through that approach.

QUADRICEPS SNIP

In the vast majority of knees, a quadriceps snip will provide just enough additional exposure to allow the revision procedure to be performed safely. Advantages of this approach include its technical ease and the fact that the surgeon's standard postoperative regimen (including weight bearing and range of motion) need not be altered.

Technique

The quadriceps snip[14,15] is an oblique apical extension of the arthrotomy across the substance of the quadriceps tendon in a proximal and lateral direction into the muscle fibers of the vastus lateralis (**Figure 5**). It is important to perform the snip in the substance of the tendon (and not more proximally, in the substance of the rectus femoris muscle) so that a strong repair is obtained. Making the snip too close to the patella itself may increase the risk for osteonecrosis of the patella secondary to vascular disruption. The snip is repaired side to side at the conclusion of the procedure, typically with heavy nonabsorbable suture. As noted above, the standard postoperative physical therapy regimen can be used with this approach.

Results

Studies that have examined the use of a quadriceps snip for exposure of the knee have all concluded that the

FIGURE 5

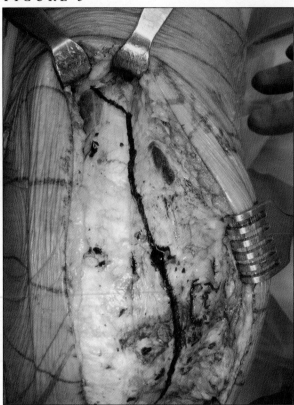

Intraoperative photograph shows a planned quadriceps snip drawn obliquely across the substance of the quadriceps tendon in a lateral and proximal direction.

complication rate is low and that the outcomes are similar to cases in which a quadriceps snip was not required. In a multicenter study of 123 knees, Barrack et al[16] found that outcomes among the 31 patients in whom a quadriceps snip was used were equivalent to outcomes in the 63 patients in whom a standard medial parapatellar arthrotomy was used. Furthermore, inferior outcomes were seen in the 14 patients who required a V-Y quadricepsplasty turndown and the 15 patients who underwent a tibial tubercle osteotomy (TTO). In a similar study by Meek et al,[17] 57 patients in whom a standard medial parapatellar approach was used were compared with 50 patients in whom a quadriceps snip was used; no differences in outcome were discernible at a minimum of 2 years. Finally, Garvin et al[15] performed strength testing on 16 patients who underwent a quadriceps snip; they found weakness in extension when compared with a normal contralateral knee but no difference when compared with a contralateral replaced knee.

V-Y QUADRICEPSPLASTY TURNDOWN

The V-Y quadricepsplasty turndown and its variants (the Coonse-Adams and patellar turndown) are rarely used in contemporary practice, being reserved for the minority of knees that are extremely stiff or ankylosed and require lengthening of the quadriceps tendon. The main impediments to the use of V-Y quadricepsplasty turndown are problems with extensor lag or weakness postoperatively and the necessity of limiting flexion postoperatively to allow for adequate healing.

Technique

In performing a V-Y quadricepsplasty turndown, the surgeon is essentially connecting a lateral retinacular release with the apex of a medial parapatellar arthrotomy proximally across the quadriceps tendon (**Figure 6**). Depending on the degree of exposure required, the incision can be continued along the lateral border of the patella and patellar tendon. If a more limited exposure that preserves the lateral geniculate vessel can be performed, this is preferable, because it may decrease the risk of devascularizing the patella and the rare but real risk of devascularizing the entire extensor mechanism with subsequent necrosis.

Closure of the V-Y quadricepsplasty turndown is done with the knee in approximately 30° of flexion, advancing the V-shaped capsular incision into a Y. Closure is performed with heavy nonabsorbable suture. Following closure, the knee is allowed to passively flex, and the amount of flexion obtained is the limit of allowable flexion (typically limited by the use of a hinged knee brace) for the first 6 weeks postoperatively. If more than 90° of flexion is obtained, the soft tissues have been advanced too far. The risk of an extensor lag will be high, and strong consideration should be given to retensioning the repair without as much soft-tissue advancement.

Results

As noted above, the study by Barrack et al[16] showed that patients who underwent V-Y quadricepsplasty turn-

FIGURE 6

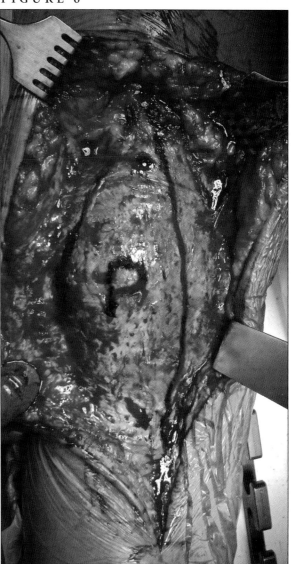

Intraoperative photograph shows a planned V-Y quadricepsplasty turndown. The apex of the medial parapatellar arthrotomy is connected with a lateral retinacular release across the quadriceps tendon. The P marks the patella.

down or TTO had inferior outcomes compared with a quadriceps snip or a standard medial parapatellar approach. When compared with the TTO group, the patients who underwent V-Y quadricepsplasty turn-

23

down had a greater increase in arc of motion, but a higher risk for extensor lag. Scott and Siliski[18] reported their results in a small series of seven knees. They described a mean increase in flexion arc of 49°; the mean extensor lag, however, was 8°. Trousdale et al[19] similarly described their results in a challenging series of 16 complex primary and revision TKAs. The mean arc of motion at a mean of 3 years was 81°. Strength testing performed on a subset of nine patients showed a trend toward decreased strength that was not significant when compared with a contralateral knee that had undergone TKA.

TIBIAL TUBERCLE OSTEOTOMY

A TTO improves exposure by essentially allowing eversion of the distal insertion of the patellar tendon and, subsequently, the patella itself.[20] Although a TTO is useful for managing the stiff knee, its greatest advantage may lie in facilitating access to the tibial canal, which can be invaluable for removing a well-fixed tibial component (particularly a long-stemmed, fully cemented component [**Figure 7**]). A TTO is more technically demanding than the soft-tissue maneuvers described previously, however, and it therefore can be more challenging for the surgeon with less experience.

Technique

The most critical aspect of a TTO is creating an osteotomy that is long enough to provide a large surface area for healing and also in a configuration that will facilitate a stable repair and not predispose to fracture of the tibial shaft. The skin incision is extended 8 to 10 cm past the insertion of the patellar tendon to expose the tibial tubercle. The osteotomy is optimally 6 to 8 cm in length and includes a bone bridge just distal to the tibial plateau that will resist proximal migration of the osteotomized tibial tubercle (**Figure 8**). If the surgeon plans on using screws for fixation of the TTO, consideration should be given to predrilling the screw holes before osteotomy creation, as this may decrease the risk of cracking or otherwise breaking the osteotomy at the time of closure. In general, the osteotomy tapers from approximately 1 cm thick proximally to 5 mm thick distally. The osteotomy is made from medial to lateral. An oscillating saw is used at first, and the cut is completed proximally and distally with either a small saw or an

FIGURE 7

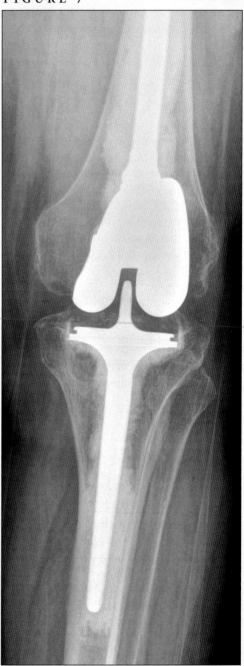

AP radiograph shows a long-stemmed, fully cemented component. Removal would be greatly facilitated by a tibial tubercle osteotomy.

FIGURE 8

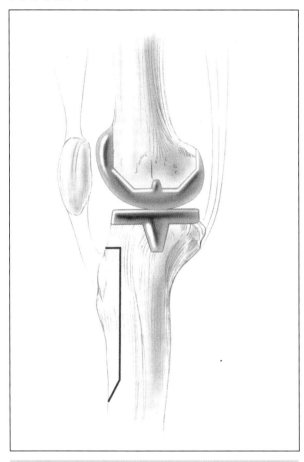

Illustration depicts a tibial tubercle osteotomy site from the lateral view. Note that the proximal extent of the osteotomy is a transverse cut and the distal extent of the osteotomy is an oblique cut. (Reproduced with permission from Nelson CL, Kim J, Lotke PA: Stiffness after total knee arthroplasty. *J Bone Joint Surg Am* 2005;87 (suppl 1:2):264-270.)

osteotome. To avoid creating a stress riser that may predispose to a tibial shaft fracture, the most distal aspect of the osteotomy should be beveled or made obliquely. The osteotomy itself is then levered open using multiple wide osteotomes, taking care to leave the soft tissues intact laterally to facilitate healing. The osteotomy is then opened as the knee is flexed, which facilitates patellar eversion. As previously suggested, if the surgeon plans on using screws for fixation at the end of the

case, consideration should be given to drilling the holes before making the osteotomy.

Following implantation of the final revision components, the osteotomy fragment is rotated back into its bed. The osteotomy should have reasonable inherent stability, particularly if a bone bridge was maintained proximally, but this may not be possible in all cases. The osteotomy can be repaired with two screws; however, if screws are used, care must be taken to avoid fracturing the bony fragment. Furthermore, the screws must be directed around the revision stem and care must be taken to avoid injuring surrounding neurovascular structures. The alternative is to use three 16-gauge stainless steel wires placed from medial to lateral via drill holes (never around the tibia itself, given the proximity of the popliteal artery to the posterior tibia) and tightened on the lateral side to minimize the risk of irritation from the knot in the wire. Specialized cables for this application are also available.

The postoperative protocol may vary by surgeon preference and the stability of the closure that is achieved. In general, active extension and straight-leg raises are avoided for 6 weeks. Similarly, flexion is typically limited to the amount obtained passively with gravity intraoperatively (but not past 90°); this is achieved by use of a hinged knee brace for 6 weeks. The brace is typically locked in extension while the patient is ambulating and weight bearing is typically allowed as tolerated, unless otherwise dictated by the tibiofemoral reconstruction.

Results

TTO was first described by Dolin,[21] but the technique was popularized by Whiteside.[20,22] The initial report of Whiteside and Ohl[20] included 71 knees followed for 1 to 5 years with no complications related to the use of a TTO for exposure. This experience was later expanded to include 136 knees (including complex primary TKAs, revisions, and revisions for infection).[22] Two fractures of the tubercle fragment were reported along with two tibial shaft fractures—one occurring following a manipulation and one in a patient with Charcot arthropathy. No nonunions were observed.

Wolff et al[23] reported a much higher rate of complications in their series of 26 TTOs, including 6 (23%) that were thought to be directly related to the exposure; osteotomy length varied, however, from only 2 cm to

9 cm. Problems included extensor mechanism disruption in 5 patients and wound healing problems in 4. Complications occurred in 3 of the 6 patients with rheumatoid arthritis. Ritter et al[24] reported two tibial shaft fractures in their initial series of nine knees; based on their experience, they suggested avoiding a transverse distal cut in favor of a gradual transition distally. Ries and Richman[25] reported on their series of 29 knees, in which the thickness of the tubercle fragment was tapered gradually from proximal to distal; they reported no fractures and only 1 case that required additional intervention to obtain bony union.

Mendes et al[26] reported serious complications in 5 patients in a series of 67 TTOs; the authors thought the approach was particularly useful in managing the infected TKA, with infection eradication achieved in 9 of 10 knees with a deep periprosthetic infection. Chalidis and Ries[27] expanded on the senior author's (M.D.R.'s) prior series in a report of 87 TTOs. Union occurred in all cases, including the 11 knees in which a repeat TTO had been performed (1 knee had undergone 3 TTOs). In addition, no differences were found among outcomes (other than an increased time to radiographic union) if the intramedullary canal was opened as part of the exposure. Young et al[28] reported on a series of 42 TTOs, which represented use of this exposure in only 4% of revision TKAs at the authors' tertiary referral center over a 12-year period. Serious complications occurred in 2 patients; both had a concomitant lateral release and TTO. The osteotomy was routinely fixed with wires, and 9 of 42 were noted to have migration of the osteotomy before bony union, although extensor lag was not a problem.

Conclusions

A medial parapatellar approach combined with a thorough anterior synovectomy will allow safe exposure for most revision TKAs. When additional exposure is required secondary to tethering of the extensor mechanism proximally, the surgeon should feel comfortable using a quadriceps snip. This maneuver is technically easy to perform and repair; no alteration in the postoperative rehabilitation is required, and the clinical results do not seem to differ if a medial parapatellar approach alone is used for exposure.

In a minority of cases, a more extensile approach will be required. If the patient has extreme stiffness and extensor mechanism lengthening is desired, a V-Y approach can be used. This approach will provide excellent exposure and is technically easy to perform; however, an extensor lag or weakness with knee extension may occur, and in rare cases, extensor mechanism necrosis can occur. This approach is not ideal for a two-stage exchange. A TTO also greatly improves exposure and is particularly useful if access to the intramedullary canal is desired for removal of a well-fixed, cemented stem. Although this technique is more technically challenging, by avoiding common pitfalls (particularly making the osteotomy long enough to provide a large surface area for healing, avoiding the creation of a stress riser in the tibial shaft), excellent results have been reported.

References

1. Markovich GD, Dorr LD, Klein NE, McPherson EJ, Vince KG: Muscle flaps in total knee arthroplasty. *Clin Orthop Relat Res* 1995;321:122-130.
2. McPherson EJ, Patzakis MJ, Gross JE, Holtom PD, Song M, Dorr LD: Infected total knee arthroplasty: Two-stage reimplantation with a gastrocnemius rotational flap. *Clin Orthop Relat Res* 1997;341:73-81.
3. Ries MD: Skin necrosis after total knee arthroplasty. *J Arthroplasty* 2002;17(4, Suppl 1):74-77.
4. Gold DA, Scott SC, Scott WN: Soft tissue expansion prior to arthroplasty in the multiply-operated knee: A new method of preventing catastrophic skin problems. *J Arthroplasty* 1996;11(5):512-521.
5. Manifold SG, Cushner FD, Craig-Scott S, Scott WN: Long-term results of total knee arthroplasty after the use of soft tissue expanders. *Clin Orthop Relat Res* 2000;380:133-139.
6. Mahomed N, McKee N, Solomon P, Lahoda L, Gross AE: Soft-tissue expansion before total knee arthroplasty in arthrodesed joints: A report of two cases. *J Bone Joint Surg Br* 1994;76(1):88-90.
7. Santore RF, Kaufman D, Robbins AJ, Dabezies EJ Jr: Tissue expansion prior to revision total knee arthroplasty. *J Arthroplasty* 1997;12(4):475-478.
8. Haertsch PA: The blood supply to the skin of the leg: A post-mortem investigation. *Br J Plast Surg* 1981;34(4):470-477.
9. Colombel M, Mariz Y, Dahhan P, Kénési C: Arterial and lymphatic supply of the knee integuments. *Surg Radiol Anat* 1998;20(1):35-40.

10. Windsor RE, Insall JN, Vince KG: Technical considerations of total knee arthroplasty after proximal tibial osteotomy. *J Bone Joint Surg Am* 1988;70(4):547-555.

11. Johnson DP, Eastwood DM: Lateral patellar release in knee arthroplasty: Effect on wound healing. *J Arthroplasty* 1992;7(Suppl):427-431.

12. Sharkey PF, Homesley HD, Shastri S, Jacoby SM, Hozack WJ, Rothman RH: Results of revision total knee arthroplasty after exposure of the knee with extensor mechanism tenolysis. *J Arthroplasty* 2004;19(6):751-756.

13. Della Valle CJ, Berger RA, Rosenberg AG: Surgical exposures in revision total knee arthroplasty. *Clin Orthop Relat Res* 2006;446:59-68.

14. Arsht SJ, Scuderi GR: The quadriceps snip for exposing the stiff knee. *J Knee Surg* 2003;16(1):55-57.

15. Garvin KL, Scuderi G, Insall JN: Evolution of the quadriceps snip. *Clin Orthop Relat Res* 1995;321:131 137.

16. Barrack RL, Smith P, Munn B, Engh G, Rorabeck C: The Ranawat Award: Comparison of surgical approaches in total knee arthroplasty. *Clin Orthop Relat Res* 1998;356:16-21.

17. Meek RM, Greidanus NV, McGraw RW, Masri BA: The extensile rectus snip exposure in revision of total knee arthroplasty. *J Bone Joint Surg Br* 2003;85(8):1120-1122.

18. Scott RD, Siliski JM: The use of a modified V-Y quadricepsplasty during total knee replacement to gain exposure and improve flexion in the ankylosed knee. *Orthopedics* 1985;8(1):45-48.

19. Trousdale RT, Hanssen AD, Rand JA, Cahalan TD: V-Y quadricepsplasty in total knee arthroplasty. *Clin Orthop Relat Res* 1993;286:48-55.

20. Whiteside LA, Ohl MD: Tibial tubercle osteotomy for exposure of the difficult total knee arthroplasty. *Clin Orthop Relat Res* 1990;260:6-9.

21. Dolin MG: Osteotomy of the tibial tubercle in total knee replacement: A technical note. *J Bone Joint Surg Am* 1983;65(5):704-706.

22. Whiteside LA: Exposure in difficult total knee arthroplasty using tibial tubercle osteotomy. *Clin Orthop Relat Res* 1995;321:32-35.

23. Wolff AM, Hungerford DS, Krackow KA, Jacobs MA: Osteotomy of the tibial tubercle during total knee replacement: A report of twenty-six cases. *J Bone Joint Surg Am* 1989;71(6):848-852.

24. Ritter MA, Carr K, Keating EM, Faris PM, Meding JB: Tibial shaft fracture following tibial tubercle osteotomy. *J Arthroplasty* 1996;11(1):117-119.

25. Ries MD, Richman JA: Extended tibial tubercle osteotomy in total knee arthroplasty. *J Arthroplasty* 1996;11(8):964-967.

26. Mendes MW, Caldwell P, Jiranek WA: The results of tibial tubercle osteotomy for revision total knee arthroplasty. *J Arthroplasty* 2004;19(2):167-174.

27. Chalidis BE, Ries MD: Does repeat tibial tubercle osteotomy or intramedullary extension affect the union rate in revision total knee arthroplasty? A retrospective study of 74 patients. *Acta Orthop* 2009;80(4):426-431.

28. Young CF, Bourne RB, Rorabeck CH: Tibial tubercle osteotomy in total knee arthroplasty surgery. *J Arthroplasty* 2008;23(3):371-375.

PROSTHESIS SELECTION: CHOOSING THE RIGHT TYPE OF CONSTRAINT

EMMANUEL THIENPONT, MD, MBA

INTRODUCTION

The aim of revision total knee arthroplasty (TKA) is to achieve excellent motion, function, and stability.[1-3] Stability in the native knee depends on several ligamentous constraints and the normal articular conformity (between the cartilage surfaces and menisci). TKA alters the function of these structures.[1,2,4] The articular surfaces (menisci and cartilage) are resected and replaced by the implant, changing the conformity of the tibiofemoral joint,[1,2,4] and ligaments are resected or released. The stability of the knee after TKA depends on the remaining soft tissues and/or the implant design.[1,2,4] Various knee prostheses are available that confer variable degrees of stability and constraint by substituting for the anatomic structures that are released and/or replaced during knee arthroplasty.[1-4]

In revision TKA, the mode of failure and the disease process also influence the quality of the bone and soft tissues.[5-7] These pathologic changes require choosing among different types of implants to suit the individual case.[8-12]

Constraint is defined in general terms as an agency that restrains movement. Morgan et al[3] defined constraint as it relates to TKA as "the effect of the elements of knee implant design that provides the stability needed to counteract forces about the knee after arthroplasty in the presence of a deficient soft-tissue envelope."

Conformity, which is the correspondence in shape and form between the femoral and tibial components, also increases implant constraint. Greater constraint stabilizes the knee by substituting for the deficient or absent ligaments.[13] In arthroplasty design, conformity and constraint are closely related.[3]

Increased constraint comes at a price because constraint transfers femorotibial joint reaction forces to the implant-bone interface, which can cause mechanical loosening.[3,5,8,10] The more the native ligaments retain their normal function and the more the implant mimics natural conformity, the less implant constraint is needed.[3,5,8,10,14]

TKA prostheses achieve constraint in two ways: through conformity and through the cam-post mechanism.[3,15] Conformity between the femoral and the tibial components will determine the amount of constraint (eg, condylar stabilizing, mobile bearing). Different types of cam-post mechanisms gradually increase the amount of constraint (from posterior stabilized [least constraint] to varus-valgus constrained [VVC] to hinged [most constraint]).

In two recent studies, instability was reported as the reason nearly 25% of all revision TKAs were performed.[1-3] Instability occurs when the available ligaments and soft-tissue structures, in combination with the prosthesis articular design and limb alignment, are unable to provide the stability necessary for adequate function in the presence of stresses transmitted across the knee joint.[1-4,16] Instability may be the result of generalized soft-tissue laxity, inadequate flexion/extension gap balancing, improper component position or alignment, or ligamentous insufficiency.[3,16-22] Such instability may occur in any plane.[23]

As a general rule, revision TKA should use a device with at least one higher level of constraint than was used in the index procedure.[7,8,10,12,14,15] This means that a unicondylar knee could be revised with a posterior cruciate ligament (PCL)–retaining knee, a PCL-retaining knee with a posterior stabilized knee, and so on.[15]

TYPES OF CONSTRAINT

Little standardization exists in the terminology used by implant manufacturers and surgeons to describe the degree of constraint provided by a particular arthroplasty design.[3,15,24] Different types of implants provide varying degrees of constraint.[3] **Table 1** lists the types of prostheses and the degree of constraint each provides.

TECHNICAL ASPECTS OF STABILITY IN REVISION TKA

In revision TKA, the stability of the previous implant and the technical aspects of the index operation should be assessed, as these factors may influence stability and limit the options available. In addition, the disease process that led to revision may influence the surgical options.

Analysis of the Index Operation

A clinical examination of the knee that assesses for stability can provide useful information regarding the degree of constraint that may be needed during revision surgery.[7,15] On the femoral side, the residual posterior condylar offset and the initial femoral component size used should be analyzed, as well as the amount of flexion of the femoral component, the alignment of the femoral component in all three planes, the joint line position, and the amount of osteolysis and bone loss. On the tibial side, the amount of posterior and eventual anterior slope, the initial tibial resection level, the frontal tibial alignment, the tibial coverage and tray position with and without stem, the type of stem (cemented or uncemented), and the stem position should be analyzed.

Analysis of the Disease Process

The disease process that led to the need for revision also can influence the revision procedure. In revisions for infection, usually a difficult approach can be expected. Even knees with articulating spacers get stiff and have limited range of motion. Often a quadriceps snip or osteotomy of the tuberosity is needed. Infection results in soft bone and thick soft tissues. Ligaments and tendinous insertions can be fragile, depending on the remaining vascularization of these tissues.

In case of aseptic loosening, more osteolysis and metal-on-metal wear can be expected than is seen on radiographs. Metallosis can be observed posteriorly on a lateral radiograph. Osteolysis remains difficult to discern on both radiographs and CT scans. In the case of fractures, the insertions of the collateral ligaments should be analyzed to understand the impact of the fracture on bone loss and stability.

The Influence of Gap Kinematics on Stability
Extension Gap

The extension gap is determined by the proximal-distal femoral position and the frontal alignment. A knee that is loose in extension can be filled with a thicker polyethylene component with an eventual release of the tighter-side collateral ligament. The amount of constraint provided by the polyethylene implant can be increased.[15] The polyethylene implant should provide sufficient medial-lateral stability. Choices range from cruciate-retaining implants (providing the least amount of stability) to hinged implants (providing maximum stability). As long as the extension gap is not bigger than the biggest polyethylene component available, the knee can be stabilized.

This technical solution faces an intrinsic problem, however: the proximalization of the joint line and the resulting low position of the patella.[25] A bigger polyethylene component requires a more proximal femoral resection and a more proximal femoral component position. As long as this resection is not proximal to the collateral ligament insertions, any type of prosthesis can be used, but the amount of proximalization will influence the implants that can be used and the clinical result.

Because the extensor mechanism will not change in length, the proximalization of the femur and a build-up

T A B L E 1 Total Knee Arthroplasty Prosthesis Types

Type of Implant	Synonyms/ Acronyms	Ligament(s) Resected	Ligament(s) Substituted
PCL-retaining	Cruciate-retaining CR TKA	ACL	None
PCL-sacrificing	Posterior cruciate–sacrificing PCS TKA	ACL-PCL	PCL by conformity
PCL-substituting	Posterior stabilized PS TKA	ACL-PCL	PCL by post and cam
ACL-PCL substituting	Bicruciate-substituting BCS TKA	ACL-PCL	ACL-PCL by post and cam
Varus-valgus constrained (VVC)	Constrained condylar knee CCK	ACL-PCL Minor laxity Collaterals	ACL-PCL by post and cam Collaterals by post and cam
Hinged	Rotating-hinge knee RHK	ACL-PCL MCL-LCL	ACL-PCL MCL-LCL

ACL = anterior cruciate ligament, BCS = bicruciate-substituting, CCK = constrained condylar knee, CR = cruciate-retaining, LCL = lateral collateral ligament, MCL = medial collateral ligament, PCL = posterior cruciate ligament, PS = posterior stabilized, TKA = total knee arthroplasty.

with a big polyethylene component will lead to a lower patellar position (patella infera).[25] In flexion, this lower position will lead to patella-post impingement in posterior stabilized and VVC implants[24] and anterior polyethylene impingement on the inferior patellar pole. This can result in limited flexion and anterior knee pain.

Frontal alignment in TKA is related to the distal femoral cut and the proximal tibial cut. Residual varus or valgus alignment without well-balanced ligaments on the opposite side can result in residual instability.

Flexion Gap
The amount of posterior tibial slope, the size of the tibial and femoral components, the interchangeability of tibial and femoral sizes and components, the flexion position of the femoral component, and the offset position of the stems will all influence the flexion gap. All of these factors are more or less related and are more difficult to control during revision surgery.

Tibial Slope
If no stem is used, different tibial slopes can be chosen. An anterior slope is rather the exception, but it could be seen when revising a TKA with a tight flexion gap. In rare cases, revising the tibial cut to a correct amount of posterior slope is sufficient. Changing the posterior slope will influence the flexion gap. With stemmed components, the stem position determines the slope of the tibial cut; in most revision systems, the correct slope is 0°. Manufacturers of most of today's revision prostheses foresee the possibility of building some slope into the polyethylene.

Size of the Tibial Component
The size of the tibial component depends on the location of the proximal tibial cut, the amount of tibial coverage, and the position of the stem. A non-offset stem may require a smaller tibial tray to avoid medial overhang. The tibial and femoral size are dependent on each other in some systems. In these size-dependent systems, a low proximal tibial cut that requires a smaller tibial component will require a smaller femoral component to be compatible. This will increase the flexion gap because the femoral size determines, through its posterior condyles, the flexion gap. Use of systems that are not size dependent can avoid this.

Flexion Position of the Femoral Component

The flexion position of the femoral component is comparable to tibial slope. Especially in revision surgery, a flexion position of the femoral component allows the use of non-offset stems to avoid an anterior femoral position. This slight flexion position increases the posterior condylar offset and stabilizes the knee in flexion. A more extended position of the femur can lead to anterior notching and overresection of the posterior condyles. The influence of a flexed femoral position on the anterior part of the tibial post has to be emphasized with regard to possible anterior post impingement or post fracture.[26]

Size of the Femoral Component

Correct sizing of the femoral component requires careful measurement. If only the anterior-posterior dimension is measured intraoperatively, failure to account for osteolysis and bone loss may lead to undersizing. The previous femoral component and the medial-lateral dimension should be measured to cross check the size. Metal wedges should be used to reconstruct the posterior bone loss to balance the flexion gap.

Especially long stems with a femoral isthmus fit will place the femoral component in a more anterior position because the natural distal femur is slightly flexed. Therefore, the anterior part will float and an overresection of the posterior condyles will be the result, leading to femoral downsizing. This anterior position is not well suited for the patella and can create instability and especially overstuffing, leading to limited flexion and anterior knee pain. Using short cemented stems and positioning the femoral component in slight flexion can help avoid this.

Offset systems are currently available that offer solutions for this problem. Usually, 360° of freedom allows the surgeon to put the femoral component in the best possible position, avoiding medial-lateral overhang and allowing anterior bony support of the component and the lowest possible posterior position. This lower posterior position fills the flexion gap, requiring less polyethylene in flexion and thus leading to a less proximal position of the femur in extension.

Polyethylene Component

The new revision systems allow the use of high-flexion polyethylene components. Thus, a too-tight flexion gap can be balanced with this design.

General Considerations

In general, posterior stabilized or VVC types of implants can improve varus-valgus instability as long as the collateral ligament instability is less than the stability of the cam-post mechanism.[15,27] Hinged implants are necessary if residual flexion gap instability is greater than the hop height of the unlinked cam-and-post mechanism.[28-32] Hinged implants also can substitute for collateral ligament absence or bone loss (bone-ligament complex).[28-32]

LEVELS OF CONSTRAINT
PCL-Retaining Implants

PCL-retaining implants, commonly known as cruciate-retaining implants, are minimally constrained prostheses that depend on an intact PCL to limit posterior translation of the tibia on the femur.[33-35]

Potential benefits of cruciate-retaining implants include less patellar clunk (soft-tissue impingement in which a soft-tissue nodule forms that can wedge into the intracondylar notch during knee flexion, causing an audible and painful "clunk"), increased quadriceps muscle strength, improved stair-climbing ability, preserved proprioceptive fibers, lowered shear forces at the tibial component–host interface, and improved preservation of bone stock on the femoral side.[3,26,33-37] In addition, cruciate-retaining implants avoid tibial post–cam-impingement or dislocation over the tibial post that can occur in posterior stabilized implants, especially in obese patients.[3,26,36,37]

In general, cruciate-retaining implants are indicated only rarely in the revision setting. Possible indications are an uncomplicated failure of a unicondylar or patellofemoral implant.[15]

PCL-Substituting Implants

In contrast to PCL-retaining implants, PCL-substituting implants have design features that limit excessive anterior-posterior tibial translation of the knee components after resection of the PCL.[3,15] The design of PCL-substituting prostheses allows controlled rollback and increases varus-valgus constraint with the substituting mechanism that improves both anterior-posterior and frontal stability.[3]

PCL-substituting implants can be divided into three types: posterior stabilized, PCL-sacrificing with ultra-congruent polyethylene components, and third-condyle knees[3] (Table 2).

TABLE 2   Types of PCL-Substituting Implants

Implant Type	Characteristics
Posterior stabilized (PS) knee	A polyethylene tibial post and a femoral cam mechanism substitute for the resected PCL.
PCL-sacrificing (PCS) knee	Increased conformity between the tibial and femoral components, often with a deep-dish design, substitutes for the resected PCL.
Third-condyle knee	The central third condyle on the femoral implant has an increased conformity with the central part of the polyethylene, substituting for the resected PCL.

PCL = posterior cruciate ligament.

Recently, interest has developed in the use of highly conforming tibial inserts to increase stability.[13] Some of these designs may eliminate the need for resection of intercondylar notch bone stock and the use of a tibial post, which has the potential to wear.[13]

Regardless of the method used to achieve posterior stability, posterior stabilized prostheses have advantages over cruciate-retaining designs, including relative ease of ligament balancing, greater versatility in the presence of different types of knee deformity, easier correction of severe deformity by eliminating a tight PCL, increased predictability in restoration of knee kinematics, improved range of motion, and potentially minimized polyethylene wear because of the option to use more congruent articular surfaces.[3,13,38-40] Furthermore, the PCL can rupture postoperatively when it is overzealously recessed intraoperatively, is tight postoperatively because of an altered joint line, or is damaged by synovitis from inflammatory arthropathy, resulting in failure.[3,38]

A potential problem with posterior stabilized implants, however, is tibial post polyethylene wear from the cam-post mechanism.[26] This problem occurs in particular with implant designs that have fixed femoral components and a posterior tibial slope.[26] Another disadvantage of posterior stabilized implants is soft-tissue impingement, including the patellar clunk syndrome. Other disadvantages include potential raising of the joint line, the need for additional bone resection to accommodate the femoral box and keel, and the risk of dislocation or instability in flexion.[3,36,41]

Despite the dissimilarities between cruciate-retaining and posterior stabilized implants, most studies have found no significant differences in function, patient satisfaction, or survivorship of the two designs in unselected patient cohorts.[42-44]

Anterior and Posterior Cruciate Ligament–Substituting Implants
Bicruciate-substituting (BCS) knees substitute for both the anterior and posterior cruciate ligaments.[45] Long-term results are not yet available.

Mobile-Bearing Implants
In mobile-bearing polyethylene designs, anterior lipping substitutes for the anterior cruciate ligament resection. The design is mobile to avoid transmission of the higher constraint because of the higher conformity with the bone-implant interface.

VVC Implants
A VVC implant has a bigger tibial post and a deeper femoral box than a posterior stabilized knee and thus provides more inherent frontal plane stability. VVC implants limit varus-valgus tilt but depend on the native ligaments for rotational stability.[23] The stem extension is important in transmitting stresses generated by the constrained articulation away from the fixation interfaces at the joint line to more normal diaphyseal bone (cementless stems) or along a broader surface area of implant-cement-bone contact (cemented stems). VVC implants may be used for both primary and revision TKA and are often helpful in the difficult primary TKA. These implants have an acceptable survival rate at intermediate follow-up, but little is known about their performance beyond 10 years.[3,27,46-48]

Drawbacks of VVC implants include the need to remove femoral intercondylar bone to accommodate the femoral box, potentially higher rates of aseptic loosening as a result of increased constraint,[43] and failure or fracture of the tibial intercondylar eminence.[3,49]

FIGURE 1

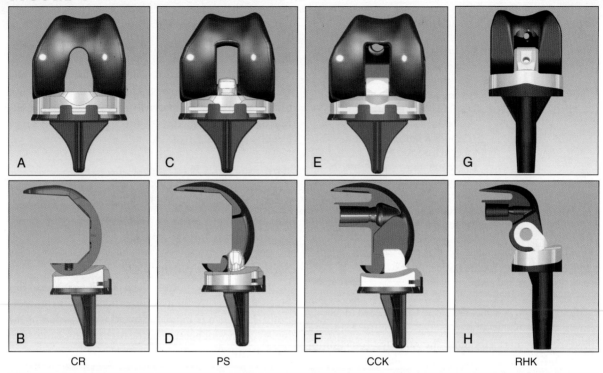

| CR | PS | CCK | RHK |

Levels of increasing constraint in total knee arthroplasty. AP (**A**) and lateral (**B**) views of a cruciate-retaining (CR) implant. AP (**C**) and lateral (**D**) views of a posterior stabilized (PS) implant. AP (**E**) and lateral (**F**) views of a constrained condylar knee (CCK) implant. AP (**G**) and lateral (**H**) views of a rotating-hinge knee (RHK) implant.

Rotating-Hinge Implants

Rotating-hinge implants are highly constrained devices, most often used for complex revision TKA performed for severe bone loss and/or complex instability and for oncologic surgery.[3,28-32] The tibial and femoral components are linked with an axle that restricts varus-valgus and translational stresses.[3,28-32] To decrease the overall amount of constraint, the tibial tray is often a mobile-bearing design.[3,28,31]

Historically, aseptic loosening and massive metal-on-metal wear were seen in uniplanar hinged knee devices because of the tremendous degree of constraint, which prohibited rotational motion.[50,51] There is still the potential drawback of forces applied across the knee being transmitted to the constraining portions of the implant or to implant-bone interfaces, leading to aseptic loosening or to unusual mechanisms of prosthesis failure.[3,8,50,52] Another drawback of rotating-hinge knee implants is that a larger bone resection is necessary to accept the housing of the implant.[3,28-32] The newer rotating-hinge knee designs make less resection of the distal femur possible (**Figure 1**).

CONSTRAINT CONSIDERATIONS

The decision about how much constraint to use is based on patient factors, the type of revision, and, potentially, the surgeon's own experience. The degree of actual or potential instability should be assessed, and the least constrained implant that will correct that instability should be chosen.

Complex Primary TKA

The use of revision components makes a complex primary TKA easier. Although a detailed discussion of this topic is beyond the scope of this chapter, primary TKA cases that may require constraint are described briefly below.[3]

Severe Varus Deformity With Intact Collateral Ligaments

In the presence of a severe varus deformity, the degree of prosthesis constraint necessary can be more important.[39] Soft-tissue releases can be difficult to control perfectly, resulting in the need for more constraint.[39,52] Potentially, an epicondylar osteotomy can achieve better results in experienced hands.[53] Both the medial approach and resection of the PCL influence the laxity of the medial compartment.[19,21] The right level of constraint will help obtain good outcomes.

Severe Valgus Deformity With Intact Collateral Ligaments

Valgus deformity can result from lateral compartment bone loss, dysplasia of the lateral condyle, medial collateral ligament (MCL) attenuation, or overcorrected high tibial osteotomy.[54-57] The preoperative assessment should be focused on the MCL. It may be normal, attenuated but present, or absent.[54-57]

The surgical treatment of knees with severe valgus deformity and intact collateral ligaments depends on the type and degree of deformity and the condition of the MCL.[3] If the MCL is present and functional, either a cruciate-retaining or posterior stabilized implant may be used. If the MCL is attenuated but present, a VVC implant may be used.[47] If the MCL is absent or associated with a rotatory instability, a rotating hinge design may be the best option.[28-32]

Patients With Rheumatoid Arthritis

Patients with rheumatoid arthritis have a higher incidence of generalized ligamentous laxity or attenuation and joint deformity.[58-60] These patients may present with severe or fixed valgus deformities requiring more constraint.[58-60]

Patients With Patellectomy

Patellectomy can cause decreased extensor mechanism power because of the loss of the fulcrum provided by the intact patella.[40,61,62] A retrospective study showed that patellectomized patients treated with posterior stabilized implants had better functional and pain scores than did patients treated with cruciate-retaining implants.[40] Bayne and Cameron[61] observed that the use of posterior stabilized devices in patients with prior patellectomies leads to better results. However, it is important to note that TKA patients with prior patellectomies generally have poorer outcomes and higher complication rates than do nonpatellectomized patients, even when posterior stabilized implants are used.[62]

Intraoperative MCL Injury

MCL injury may occur intraoperatively. In one series of 600 consecutive knees with either varus or neutral alignment treated with primary TKA, 16 knees (2.7%) sustained an inadvertent complete MCL injury intraoperatively.[63] The injuries were either midsubstance disruptions or complete avulsions of the ligament from bone during the procedure.[63] Although this can occur in patients with normal body mass,[63] Winiarsky et al[64] reported that intraoperative MCL injury occurred far more frequently in morbidly obese patients.

Historically, iatrogenic MCL injury has been treated using VVC implants, although evidence-based support for this approach is lacking because of the relative infrequency of the complication.[3,4,46,48] In one series, 16 knees were successfully treated primarily with reattachment or repair and bracing. No patient required bracing beyond the initial 6-week period, and no patient demonstrated coronal plane instability.[63]

Complex Instability

It is not possible to anticipate every pattern of deformity that might be present in the context of primary TKA, especially in the multiply operated patient.[25] Chronic anterior cruciate ligament or MCL instability can cause surprising residual medial laxity in flexion. In such cases, the surgeon may have to decide between opposite-side ligament release, ligament advancement, a VVC implant, or, in the most severe cases, a rotating-hinge prosthesis.

Revision TKA

Different types of constraint are appropriate in different revision TKA settings, from cruciate-retaining to hinged prostheses. Table 3 lists the types of constraint indicated in various situations.

TABLE 3 Types of Constraint Indicated in Revision Total Knee Arthroplasty

Type of Knee Being Revised	Appropriate Constraint Choices
Unicondylar knee	Cruciate-retaining PCL-sacrificing Posterior stabilized
Failed primary TKA	PCL-sacrificing Posterior stabilized Varus-valgus constrained Rotating-hinge
Failed revision TKA	Varus-valgus constrained Rotating-hinge

PCL = posterior cruciate ligament, TKA = total knee arthroplasty.

Complicated Scenarios

Other patients may benefit from constrained or hinged implants. These include elderly patients with comminuted distal femur fractures or periprosthetic fracture nonunion, patients with extensor mechanism disruptions and unstable knees, and patients with marked bone loss or tumors.[3]

Other Factors That Influence Implant Choice

Surgeons should also consider the following factors when selecting a prosthesis. The technical possibilities and limitations of a certain design of implant will decide the amount of constraint that is indicated.

Technical Features

The following technical features are desirable in an implant.

- It is always desirable to be able to change to a different type of constraint within the same system during surgery (eg, from posterior stabilized to VVC or even to a hinged design). This avoids having to have multiple implant systems available in case more constraint than expected is necessary.
- An implant that allows for interchangeability among various femoral and tibial component sizes is desirable because it does not limit the surgeon's sizing choice. A small tibial component can be used with any size femoral component without the need for higher constraint.
- An implant with offset stems avoids tibial down-sizing to eliminate medial overhang on the tibial side and avoids a femoral anterior position with an increased flexion gap.
- An implant with high-flexion polyethylene options allows balancing of the flexion gap if it is too tight.
- An implant with full choice between cemented and uncemented stems of different lengths allows the surgeon to adapt the reconstruction to the surgical conditions of the case.
- An implant with a mobile-bearing design for the more constrained types of implants is desirable because this design avoids transmitting the higher constraint to the bone-implant interface, which could result in loosening.

MCL Repair or Reconstruction

In some indications, the surgeon can decrease the type of constraint needed by augmenting the stability of the available ligaments. The collateral ligaments are especially useful for augmenting stability, if the surgeon has the technical skill required for this type of procedure.

Advancement, imbrication, or allograft reconstruction of the MCL may be done to treat medial-side laxity in conjunction with a VVC implant.[65] Advantages of imbrication or advancement include the potential for increased component survivorship because stress transmission to the fixation surfaces is decreased and allograft tissue, as would be needed for ligament reconstruction, is not required.[3] Disadvantages of this technique include the potential for late attenuation or rupture of the repair and the difficulty of getting satisfactory ligament balance in both flexion and extension, largely because there is no true isometric point for the MCL that exists throughout the range of motion.[3]

Advantages of ligament reconstruction include that it decreases the amount of implant constraint necessary. Disadvantages include the technical difficulty of flexion-extension ligament balancing, increased surgical time, and donor-site morbidity associated with autografts.[3]

CONCLUSIONS

The amount of constraint to be used in a particular revision is an important element of preoperative planning and is partially a preoperative decision. Using an implant with insufficient constraint risks early failure from instability, whereas using a device that has more constraint than is necessary can predispose the patient to aseptic loosening and bone loss in the long run.[3] Clinical factors such as the underlying disease, severe coronal plane deformity, collateral ligament deficiencies, or severe bone loss may influence the decision regarding the degree of constraint to be used. As a general rule, the least constrained implant that provides satisfactory joint stability should be chosen. In experienced hands, soft-tissue repair or ligament reconstruction may help decrease the level of constraint needed. Constraint should not be a substitute for good preoperative planning, surgical technique, or knowledge of basic TKA gap mechanics.

REFERENCES

1. Fehring TK, Odum S, Griffin WL, Mason JB, Nadaud M: Early failures in total knee arthroplasty. *Clin Orthop Relat Res* 2001;392:315-318.

2. Sharkey PF, Hozack WJ, Rothman RH, Shastri S, Jacoby SM: Insall Award paper: Why are total knee arthroplasties failing today? *Clin Orthop Relat Res* 2002;404:7-13.

3. Morgan H, Battista V, Leopold SS: Constraint in primary total knee arthroplasty. *J Am Acad Orthop Surg* 2005;13(8):515-524.

4. Cameron HU, Hunter GA: Failure in total knee arthroplasty: Mechanisms, revisions, and results. *Clin Orthop Relat Res* 1982;170:141-146.

5. Cuckler JM: Revision total knee arthroplasty: How much constraint is necessary? *Orthopedics* 1995;18(9): 932-933, 936.

6. Gallagher JA, Bourne RB: The role of implant constraint in revision total knee replacement: Striking the balance. *Orthopedics* 2004;27(9):995-996.

7. Gustke KA: Preoperative planning for revision total knee arthroplasty: Avoiding chaos. *J Arthroplasty* 2005;20(4, Suppl 2):37-40.

8. McAuley JP, Engh GA: Constraint in total knee arthroplasty: When and what? *J Arthroplasty* 2003;18(3, Suppl 1):51-54.

9. Insall JN: Constraint in TKA: Elderly patient, elderly surgeon? *Orthopedics* 1999;22(9):885-886.

10. Laskin RS: Articular constraint: Use only what you need. *Orthopedics* 2003;26(9):975-976.

11. Naudie DD, Rorabeck CH: Managing instability in total knee arthroplasty with constrained and linked implants. *Instr Course Lect* 2004;53:207-215.

12. Scuderi GR: Revision total knee arthroplasty: How much constraint is enough? *Clin Orthop Relat Res* 2001;392:300-305.

13. Hofmann AA, Tkach TK, Evanich CJ, Camargo MP: Posterior stabilization in total knee arthroplasty with use of an ultracongruent polyethylene insert. *J Arthroplasty* 2000;15(5):576-583.

14. Sculco TP: The role of constraint in total knee arthroplasty. *J Arthroplasty* 2006;21(4, Suppl 1):54-56.

15. Lombardi AV Jr, Berend KR: Posterior cruciate ligament-retaining, posterior stabilized, and varus/valgus posterior stabilized constrained articulations in total knee arthroplasty. *Instr Course Lect* 2006;55:419-427.

16. Rorabeck CH: The unstable total knee: Causes and cures. *Knee* 2001;8(3):179-186.

17. Vince KG, Abdeen A, Sugimori T: The unstable total knee arthroplasty: Causes and cures. *J Arthroplasty* 2006;21(4, Suppl 1):44-49.

18. Clarke HD, Scuderi GR: Flexion instability in primary total knee replacement. *J Knee Surg* 2003;16(2):123-128.

19. Krackow KA, Mihalko WM: The effect of medial release on flexion and extension gaps in cadaveric knees: Implications for soft-tissue balancing in total knee arthroplasty. *Am J Knee Surg* 1999;12(4):222-228.

20. Martin JW, Whiteside LA: The influence of joint line position on knee stability after condylar knee arthroplasty. *Clin Orthop Relat Res* 1990;259:146-156.

21. Mihalko WM, Krackow KA: Posterior cruciate ligament effects on the flexion space in total knee arthroplasty. *Clin Orthop Relat Res* 1999;360:243-250.

22. Saeki K, Mihalko WM, Patel V, et al: Stability after medial collateral ligament release in total knee arthroplasty. *Clin Orthop Relat Res* 2001;392:184-189.

23. Whiteside LA, Kasselt MR, Haynes DW: Varus-valgus and rotational stability in rotationally unconstrained total knee arthroplasty. *Clin Orthop Relat Res* 1987;219:147-157.

24. Verborgt O, Victor J: Post impingement in posterior stabilised total knee arthroplasty. *Acta Orthop Belg* 2004;70(1):46-50.

25. Yoshii I, Whiteside LA, White SE, Milliano MT: Influence of prosthetic joint line position on knee kinematics and patellar position. *J Arthroplasty* 1991;6(2): 169-177.

26. Callaghan JJ, O'Rourke MR, Goetz DD, Schmalzried TP, Campbell PA, Johnston RC: Tibial post impingement in posterior-stabilized total knee arthroplasty. *Clin Orthop Relat Res* 2002;404:83-88.

27. Hartford JM, Goodman SB, Schurman DJ, Knoblick G: Complex primary and revision total knee arthroplasty using the condylar constrained prosthesis: An average 5-year follow-up. *J Arthroplasty* 1998;13(4):380-387.

28. Barrack RL, Lyons TR, Ingraham RQ, Johnson JC: The use of a modular rotating hinge component in salvage revision total knee arthroplasty. *J Arthroplasty* 2000;15(7):858-866.

29. Rand JA, Chao EY, Stauffer RN: Kinematic rotating-hinge total knee arthroplasty. *J Bone Joint Surg Am* 1987;69(4):489-497.

30. Westrich GH, Mollano AV, Sculco TP, Buly RL, Laskin RS, Windsor R: Rotating hinge total knee arthroplasty in severly affected knees. *Clin Orthop Relat Res* 2000;379:195-208.

31. Barrack RL: Evolution of the rotating hinge for complex total knee arthroplasty. *Clin Orthop Relat Res* 2001;392:292-299.

32. Springer BD, Hanssen AD, Sim FH, Lewallen DG: The kinematic rotating hinge prosthesis for complex knee arthroplasty. *Clin Orthop Relat Res* 2001;392:283-291.

33. Banks SA, Hodge WA: Implant design affects knee arthroplasty kinematics during stair-stepping. *Clin Orthop Relat Res* 2004;426:187-193.

34. Dennis DA, Komistek RD, Colwell CE Jr, et al: In vivo anteroposterior femorotibial translation of total knee arthroplasty: A multicenter analysis. *Clin Orthop Relat Res* 1998;356:47-57.

35. Kanekasu K, Banks SA, Honjo S, Nakata O, Kato H: Fluoroscopic analysis of knee arthroplasty kinematics during deep flexion kneeling. *J Arthroplasty* 2004;19(8):998-1003.

36. Gidwani S, Langkamer VG: Recurrent dislocation of a posterior-stabilized prosthesis: A series of three cases. *Knee* 2001;8(4):317-320.

37. Most E, Zayontz S, Li G, Otterberg E, Sabbag K, Rubash HE: Femoral rollback after cruciate-retaining and stabilizing total knee arthroplasty. *Clin Orthop Relat Res* 2003;410:101-113.

38. Waslewski GL, Marson BM, Benjamin JB: Early, incapacitating instability of posterior cruciate ligament-retaining total knee arthroplasty. *J Arthroplasty* 1998;13(7):763-767.

39. Laskin RS: The Insall Award: Total knee replacement with posterior cruciate ligament retention in patients with a fixed varus deformity. *Clin Orthop Relat Res* 1996;331:29-34.

40. Paletta GA Jr, Laskin RS: Total knee arthroplasty after a previous patellectomy. *J Bone Joint Surg Am* 1995;77(11):1708-1712.

41. Beight JL, Yao B, Hozack WJ, Hearn SL, Booth RE Jr: The patellar "clunk" syndrome after posterior stabilized total knee arthroplasty. *Clin Orthop Relat Res* 1994;299:139-142.

42. Clark CR, Rorabeck CH, MacDonald S, MacDonald D, Swafford J, Cleland D: Posterior-stabilized and cruciate-retaining total knee replacement: A randomized study. *Clin Orthop Relat Res* 2001;392:208-212.

43. Forster MC: Survival analysis of primary cemented total knee arthroplasty: Which designs last? *J Arthroplasty* 2003;18(3):265-270.

44. Becker MW, Insall JN, Faris PM: Bilateral total knee arthroplasty: One cruciate retaining and one cruciate substituting. *Clin Orthop Relat Res* 1991;271:122-124.

45. Victor J, Bellemans J: Physiologic kinematics as a concept for better flexion in TKA. *Clin Orthop Relat Res* 2006;452:53-58.

46. Donaldson WF III, Sculco TP, Insall JN, Ranawat CS: Total condylar III knee prosthesis: Long-term follow-up study. *Clin Orthop Relat Res* 1988;226:21-28.

47. Easley ME, Insall JN, Scuderi GR, Bullek DD: Primary constrained condylar knee arthroplasty for the arthritic valgus knee. *Clin Orthop Relat Res* 2000;380:58-64.

48. Lachiewicz PF, Falatyn SP: Clinical and radiographic results of the Total Condylar III and Constrained Condylar total knee arthroplasty. *J Arthroplasty* 1996;11(8):916-922.

49. McPherson EJ, Vince KG: Breakage of a Total Condylar III knee prosthesis: A case report. *J Arthroplasty* 1993;8(5):561-563.

50. Wang CJ, Wang HE: Early catastrophic failure of rotating hinge total knee prosthesis. *J Arthroplasty* 2000;15(3):387-391.

51. Pour AE, Parvizi J, Slenker N, Purtill JJ, Sharkey PF: Rotating hinged total knee replacement: Use with caution. *J Bone Joint Surg Am* 2007;89(8):1735-1741.

52. Teeny SM, Krackow KA, Hungerford DS, Jones M: Primary total knee arthroplasty in patients with severe varus deformity: A comparative study. *Clin Orthop Relat Res* 1991;273:19-31.

53. Engh GA, Ammeen D: Results of total knee arthroplasty with medial epicondylar osteotomy to correct varus deformity. *Clin Orthop Relat Res* 1999;367:141-148.

54. Whiteside LA: Selective ligament release in total knee arthroplasty of the knee in valgus. *Clin Orthop Relat Res* 1999;367:130-140.

55. Miyasaka KC, Ranawat CS, Mullaji A: 10- to 20-year followup of total knee arthroplasty for valgus deformities. *Clin Orthop Relat Res* 1997;345:29-37.

56. Whiteside LA: Correction of ligament and bone defects in total arthroplasty of the severely valgus knee. *Clin Orthop Relat Res* 1993;288:234-245.

57. Krackow KA, Jones MM, Teeny SM, Hungerford DS: Primary total knee arthroplasty in patients with fixed valgus deformity. *Clin Orthop Relat Res* 1991;273:9-18.

58. Archibeck MJ, Berger RA, Barden RM, et al: Posterior cruciate ligament-retaining total knee arthroplasty in patients with rheumatoid arthritis. *J Bone Joint Surg Am* 2001;83-A(8):1231-1236.

59. Hanyu T, Murasawa A, Tojo T: Survivorship analysis of total knee arthroplasty with the kinematic prosthesis in patients who have rheumatoid arthritis. *J Arthroplasty* 1997;12(8):913-919.

60. Laskin RS, O'Flynn HM: The Insall Award: Total knee replacement with posterior cruciate ligament retention in rheumatoid arthritis: Problems and complications. *Clin Orthop Relat Res* 1997;345:24-28.

61. Bayne O, Cameron HU: Total knee arthroplasty following patellectomy. *Clin Orthop Relat Res* 1984;186:112-114.

62. Cameron HU, Hu C, Vyamont D: Posterior stabilized knee prosthesis for total knee replacement in patients with prior patellectomy. *Can J Surg* 1996;39(6):469-473.

63. Leopold SS, McStay C, Klafeta K, Jacobs JJ, Berger RA, Rosenberg AG: Primary repair of intraoperative disruption of the medical collateral ligament during total knee arthroplasty. *J Bone Joint Surg Am* 2001;83-A(1):86-91.

64. Winiarsky R, Barth P, Lotke P: Total knee arthroplasty in morbidly obese patients. *J Bone Joint Surg Am* 1998;80(12):1770-1774.

65. Healy WL, Iorio R, Lemos DW: Medial reconstruction during total knee arthroplasty for severe valgus deformity. *Clin Orthop Relat Res* 1998;356:161-169.

PERIPROSTHETIC KNEE INFECTIONS: CONTRIBUTING FACTORS

NITIN GOYAL, MD

JAMES J. PURTILL, MD

INTRODUCTION

Surgical-site infection is one of the most common and devastating complications after total joint arthroplasty, with a reported prevalence of 0.5% to 3%.[1-4] The reported prevalence of infection after total knee arthroplasty (TKA) is higher than for total hip arthroplasty;[1-4] the infection rate after revision TKA may be as high as 4% to 8%.[5-10] Infection following TKA represents a significant challenge for both the surgeon and the patient. Additionally, the estimated cost for treatment of an infected TKA may be more than $60,000.[11] Fortunately, improved preventive efforts with prophylactic antibiotics, laminar airflow rooms, body exhaust suits, and increasingly swift diagnosis and management have reduced infection rates.[3] This decrease has been eclipsed, however, by the extraordinary increase in the number of TKAs done yearly in the United States. Current research continues to focus on improving the diagnosis of periprosthetic joint infection and effectively tailoring the treatment of each patient, considering medical comorbidities, the specific infectious organism, the local bone stock, and soft-tissue coverage.

The risk of infection after TKA is directly correlated to a variety of factors that may be divided into those related to the host, the organism, and the environment. The risk of infection of the wound is directly related to the local wound, the number and virulence of the bacteria in or near the wound, and the host's ability to mount an inflammatory response and fight the bacteria. The methodology of prevention must focus on optimizing the local wound environment, maximizing the nutritional and immunologic status of the patient, and minimizing bacterial contamination (reducing the number of colony-forming units in or near the wound). This requires a multifaceted approach during the preoperative, intraoperative, and postoperative stages.

HOST FACTORS

The Cierny-Mader classification[12] of osteomyelitis may be used to classify infectious host types in TKA infection (**Table 1**). This system classifies the patient as an A, B, or C host. An A host is a patient with normal physiologic, immunologic, and metabolic status. A B host is locally compromised, systemically compromised, or both. When the morbidity of treatment is worse than the disease itself, the patient is classified as a C host. Host factors are chiefly related to containment of the infection. A type B host does not contain infection as well as a type A host, and infection in the type B host will prove more complex to treat. This classification system provides a useful framework for analyzing how host factors directly relate to the effectiveness of any infection treatment and to the ability of the host to fight any bacterial contamination.

Certain medical comorbidities can significantly affect the infection rate in patients undergoing total joint arthro-

Neither of the following authors nor any immediate family member has received anything of value from or owns stock in a commercial company or institution related directly or indirectly to the subject of this chapter: Dr. Goyal and Dr. Purtill.

TABLE 1 Cierny-Mader Osteomyelitis Staging Classification

Host Type	Description
A	Normal physiologic, immunologic, and metabolic status
B	Local compromise, systemic compromise, or systemic and local compromise
C	Treatment worse than disease

FIGURE 1

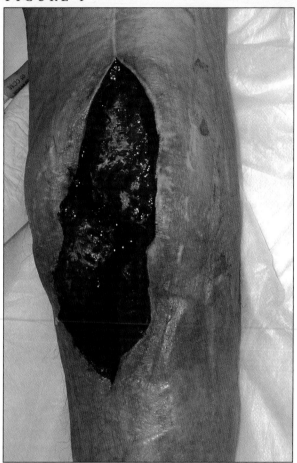

Intraoperative photograph shows the knee of a patient with rheumatoid arthritis who underwent total knee arthroplasty. Postoperative hematoma and delayed wound healing developed, leading to wound dehiscence and deep infection.

plasty. Wound healing and the ability to combat foreign organisms may be altered in patients with certain disease states. In particular, multiple investigators have found that the propensity to develop infection following joint arthroplasty surgery is increased in patients with rheumatoid arthritis (RA).[6,13-19] Wilson et al[20] reported on 67 infections in a series of more than 4,000 TKAs in which they found infection was 2.5 times more likely to develop in the knees of patients with RA than in patients with osteoarthritis. The authors also demonstrated that men with RA were at higher risk of infection than women with RA. This increased infection risk in patients with RA may be due to a high rate of delayed or unsuccessful wound healing[21] (**Figure 1**). In addition, patients with RA have been reported to have decreased neutrophil function, which may result in weakened host resistance to infection.[22]

Multiple studies have demonstrated an association between the use of corticosteroids and an increased risk of infection in patients who have RA.[16,23,24] The need for perioperative corticosteroids may be indicative of the severity of the inflammatory process in the RA patient.[20]

Patients with diabetes mellitus are prone to infection after surgical procedures (**Figure 2**). This may be a result of impaired macrophage phagocytosis as well as poor host-defense mechanisms, which has been illustrated in multiple experimental models.[25-27] Several investigators have also reported an association between diabetes mellitus and increased risk of wound complications and deep infection. For example, in a report of more than 17,000 primary TKAs, 59 knees were found to have early wound complications. The only variable associated with this early wound complication rate was a diagnosis of diabetes mellitus.[28]

Diminished nutritional status also has been demonstrated to have a substantial impact on the risk of postop-erative complications. A preoperative lymphocyte count of fewer than 1,500 cells/mm^3 (a measure of nutritional deficiency) correlated with a five times greater frequency of major wound complications following total joint arthroplasty. In addition, an albumin level of less than 3.5 g/dL (a second measure of malnutrition) was associated with a seven times greater frequency of wound complications.[29] Patients with an albumin level less than 3.9 g/dL have been shown to be twice as likely to require prolonged hos-

FIGURE 2

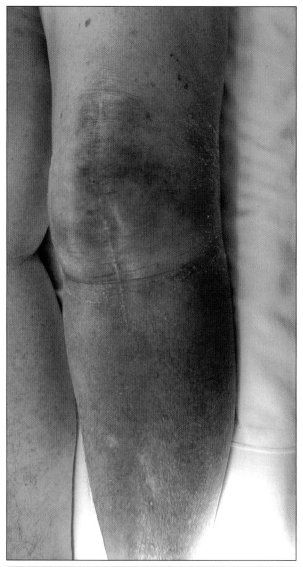

Clinical photograph of the knee of a patient with brittle diabetes who underwent total knee arthroplasty. Early postoperative severe cellulitis and subsequent deep infection developed.

pitalization (>15 days) when compared with patients with an albumin level of 3.9 g/dL or greater.[30]

Immunocompromised patients have a higher risk of complications after total joint arthroplasty. Patients who are human immunodeficiency virus (HIV) positive have been shown to have a deep infection rate as high as 30% and a rate of complications that require repeat operation of 60%.[31] Patients and surgeons need to be aware of these high complication rates so that a forthright discussion can take place regarding the expectations and risk-benefit ratio before any surgical intervention.

Obesity has been shown to increase the risk of postoperative infection.[32] Obesity (defined as body mass index > 30 kg/m^2) has been demonstrated to be an independent risk factor for prolonged wound drainage after total joint arthroplasty, and it has been identified as an independent risk factor for infection following TKA.[33]

Ectopic sources of infection also must be evaluated preoperatively in patients undergoing total joint arthroplasty. Patients should be evaluated for dental caries, genitourinary tract infections, pulmonary infections, and skin wounds or ulcers because these conditions may be sources of bacterial seeding of a prosthetic implant in the early postoperative period. In a review of more than 4,000 primary TKAs, patients who had undergone a previous knee operation had a more than four times higher risk of joint infection compared with patients who had not undergone a prior surgical procedure around the knee.[20] A study of TKA in patients with a history of native knee septic arthritis or osteomyelitis demonstrated that a recurrent deep infection developed in 1 in 20 patients.[34] The authors concluded that with careful preoperative workup, intraoperative evaluation, and the use of antibiotic-impregnated cement, TKA can provide good pain relief, functional improvement, and an acceptably low rate of deep prosthetic infection in patients with prior joint sepsis or osteomyelitis.

The identification of patients who are at a higher risk for infection following TKA is critical in providing both the patient and the surgeon with accurate information about the risks and benefits of the procedure and a realistic expectation of outcomes. Additionally, a detailed evaluation and risk assessment is vital in ensuring optimal medical and surgical management both intraoperatively and postoperatively for patients who are predisposed to infection.

PROPHYLACTIC ANTIBIOTICS
Increased bacterial load (contamination) and subsequent deep infection most commonly arise from either skin or airborne sources.[35,36] The most common organisms that result in deep wound infection in orthopaedic

　　　　　　　　　　　　　　43

surgery are *Staphylococcus aureus* and coagulase-negative *Staphylococcus* species, specifically *S epidermidis*.[36-39] Based on these infectious organism patterns, either cefazolin or cefuroxime should be used as a preoperative prophylactic antibiotic for hip and knee arthroplasty.[37,40-42] The first-generation cephalosporins have been studied extensively and found to have excellent in vivo activity against *Staphylococcus* and *Streptococcus* species with a long half-life and good tissue penetration. Vancomycin or clindamycin may be used for patients with a history of adverse reactions to the β-lactam group of antibiotics. No level I evidence exists comparing the efficacy of vancomycin with that of clindamycin for prophylaxis against deep infection in orthopaedic surgery; thus, no preference is made between the two. In randomized clinical trials comparing the effectiveness of vancomycin to first-generation cephalosporins (cefazolin/cefuroxime) for the prevention of postoperative infection, no benefit was demonstrated in the vancomycin group, although there was a lower incidence of methicillin-resistant *S aureus* infections in the vancomycin group.[43,44]

Antibiotics should preferably be administered within 60 minutes before incision.[45-47] To improve compliance, antibiotic administration should be part of the anesthesiology protocol, and, preferably, as a safeguard, a verification of administration should be part of the "time out" at the start of the procedure. An additional dose of antibiotics may be given intraoperatively if significant blood loss occurs during the procedure or if the procedure extends longer than one to two times the half-life of the antibiotic.[48,49] Current recommendations include prophylactic antibiotic administration in total joint arthroplasty patients for up to 24 hours postoperatively. Longer antibiotic prophylaxis is currently not supported by the literature consensus or Centers for Disease Control (CDC) recommendations.[38,50]

OPERATING ROOM ENVIRONMENT

Certain operating room environment details related to infection are perceived as modifiable and are often addressed at length (eg, careful draping), but other factors are frequently overlooked. Wound contamination in the operating room occurs either by direct fallout or by contact with contaminated instruments or gloves. To effectively contain environmental contamination of surgical wounds in total joint arthroplasty, it is important to understand that operating room personnel are thought to be the greatest source of airborne bacteria. The quantity of environmental bacteria in the operating room is directly related to the number of personnel present and the amount of bacteria each person sheds.[51] Approximately 30% of operating room personnel are carriers for *S aureus*. Most people shed between 1,000 and 10,000 bacteria per minute, but up to 13% of men, 5% of postmenopausal women, and 1% of premenopausal women are so-called "dispersers," shedding more than 10,000 bacteria per minute.[51] A sterile body exhaust is the most effective means of preventing contamination from bacterial shedding, but this requires a full "space suit," which is not preferable or practical for the anesthesia team or unscrubbed circulating nursing staff. In 1999, Ritter[52] evaluated contamination levels in the operating room environment in a variety of circumstances and found that the amount of bacteria in the operating room could be decreased effectively by reducing the number of personnel, using inclusive gowning, minimizing operating room time, and using an environmental control system such as laminar airflow.

Sterilized instrumentation and devices are assumed to remain sterile throughout a procedure until used, but multiple studies have shown that instruments become contaminated during the course of a procedure if they are left open and exposed to the operating room environment. In 2008, Dalstrom et al[53] evaluated open, sterilized instrument trays in a controlled operating room environment and found that culture positivity related directly to the duration of open, uncovered exposure. The authors reported a culture-positive rate for open, uncovered trays of 22% at 2 hours and 30% at 4 hours. They also found that the simple step of covering the surgical tray with a sterile towel significantly reduced the contamination risk. Ritter[52] published similar results in 1999, stating that more than one half of all untouched instruments in conventional operating rooms are contaminated after 3 hours of surgical time.

Another noteworthy source of contamination in orthopaedic surgery, specifically total joint arthroplasty, is the splash basin used to soak surgical instruments. With its large exposed surface area, the splash basin may serve as a perfect settling place for micro-

FIGURE 3

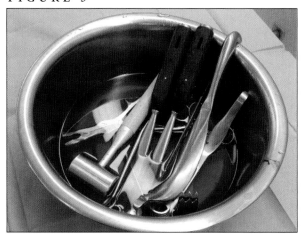

An example of a splash basin used to soak surgical instruments in total joint arthroplasty.

FIGURE 4

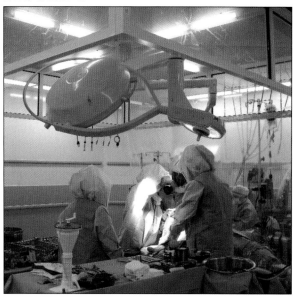

Photograph shows an operating room equipped with laminar airflow.

bial matter and airborne particulates (**Figure 3**). Baird et al[54] evaluated splash basin contamination during orthopaedic operations and found a culture-positive rate of 74%, with multiple organisms found in 59% of the basins. In a similar study, Andersson et al[55] found that 62% of sterile open irrigation solutions became contaminated during procedures lasting 1 hour or longer.

Suction tips used in total hip arthroplasty have been evaluated. Strange-Vognsen and Klareskov[56] found that 55% of suction tips were culture-positive. A similar study by Greenough[57] demonstrated that time-dependent contamination of suction tips occurred in total hip arthroplasty, with a 37% contamination rate when one suction tip was used for the duration of an operation.

Modern orthopaedic operating room design has evolved in response to the need to reduce bacterial contamination. Charnley and Eftekhar[58] investigated the penetration of gown material by organisms from the surgeon's body; on the basis of their findings, exhaust suit systems were developed. Ritter[52] confirmed that body exhaust suits resulted in a 38% reduction in environmental bacteria compared with plastic wraparound gowns and a 69% reduction compared with scrub clothes.

Surgical draping must exclude bacteria from the surgical field. Blom et al[59] evaluated seven different types of surgical drapes for bacterial penetration. Woven drapes were shown to have rapid bacterial penetration, whereas nonwoven, disposable drapes did not. Complete disinfection of the skin with surgical skin preparation is nearly impossible because of the hair follicles and sebaceous glands that harbor most of the bacteria, but using skin barriers to prevent lateral migration of skin bacteria can significantly reduce the contamination during surgery. Johnston et al[60] demonstrated that plastic drapes impregnated with slow-release iodophor can eliminate bacterial colonization on the skin for up to 3 hours. Additionally, iodophor-impregnated plastic adhesive drapes have been demonstrated to reduce deep wound contamination by skin organisms almost tenfold in hip surgery.[61]

Laminar airflow rooms (**Figure 4**) are often implemented for total joint arthroplasty surgery. High-efficiency particulate air filters remove 99.97% of all particles 0.3 μm or more in diameter. In addition, because the air flows with uniform velocity parallel to the patient, the number of bacterial colony–forming units in the surgical field is reduced.[62] The use of laminar airflow operating rooms has reduced operating room airborne bacterial contamination and significantly decreased infection rates.[62]

Ultraviolet lighting is an alternative approach; it reduces surgical infection by killing bacteria in the surgical field. Ritter et al[63] compared ultraviolet lighting with horizontal laminar airflow in joint arthroplasty surgery. A series of 5,980 total joint arthroplasty procedures performed by the same surgeon were studied. The first 1,071 procedures were performed in a horizontal laminar airflow room; the following 4,909 procedures were performed with ultraviolet lighting. A 3.1 times greater risk of infection was found for procedures performed with horizontal laminar airflow. Ultraviolet lighting has had limited use, however, because of concerns regarding exposure of the operating room personnel and the patient to the potentially harmful effects of the light. Ultraviolet light is inexpensive and may be an excellent alternative to laminar airflow systems as long as proper exposure precautions are observed.

CONCLUSIONS

Infection after TKA is a devastating complication. Treatment of the patient with an infected prosthetic joint requires prolonged hospitalization and intravenous antibiotic therapy. Multiple surgical procedures may be necessary, which can lead to significant morbidity for the patient. Thorough preoperative patient evaluation for host factors and medical comorbidities is necessary to optimize surgical outcome with regard to infection. Meticulous attention to detail in the operating room is necessary to limit potential sources of bacterial contamination and optimize the surgical environment.

REFERENCES

1. Hanssen AD, Rand JA: Evaluation and treatment of infection at the site of a total hip or knee arthroplasty. *Instr Course Lect* 1999;48:111-122.

2. Joseph TN, Chen AL, Di Cesare PE: Use of antibiotic-impregnated cement in total joint arthroplasty. *J Am Acad Orthop Surg* 2003;11(1):38-47.

3. Peersman G, Laskin R, Davis J, Peterson M: Infection in total knee replacement: A retrospective review of 6489 total knee replacements. *Clin Orthop Relat Res* 2001;392:15-23.

4. Durbhakula SM, Czajka J, Fuchs MD, Uhl RL: Spacer endoprosthesis for the treatment of infected total hip arthroplasty. *J Arthroplasty* 2004;19(6):760-767.

5. Bengtson S, Knutson K: The infected knee arthroplasty: A 6-year follow-up of 357 cases. *Acta Orthop Scand* 1991;62(4):301-311.

6. Grogan TJ, Dorey F, Rollins J, Amstutz HC: Deep sepsis following total knee arthroplasty: Ten-year experience at the University of California at Los Angeles Medical Center. *J Bone Joint Surg Am* 1986;68(2):226-234.

7. Johnson DP, Bannister GC: The outcome of infected arthroplasty of the knee. *J Bone Joint Surg Br* 1986;68(2):289-291.

8. Rand JA, Bryan RS, Morrey BF, Westholm F: Management of infected total knee arthroplasty. *Clin Orthop Relat Res* 1986;205:75-85.

9. Springer BD, Lee GC, Osmon D, Haidukewych GJ, Hanssen AD, Jacofsky DJ: Systemic safety of high-dose antibiotic-loaded cement spacers after resection of an infected total knee arthroplasty. *Clin Orthop Relat Res* 2004;427:47-51.

10. Windsor RE: Management of total knee arthroplasty infection. *Orthop Clin North Am* 1991;22(3):531-538.

11. Hebert CK, Williams RE, Levy RS, Barrack RL: Cost of treating an infected total knee replacement. *Clin Orthop Relat Res* 1996;331:140-145.

12. Cierny G III, Mader JT, Penninck JJ: A clinical staging system for adult osteomyelitis. *Clin Orthop Relat Res* 2003;414:7-24.

13. D'Ambrosia RD, Shoji H, Heater R: Secondarily infected total joint replacements by hematogenous spread. *J Bone Joint Surg Am* 1976;58(4):450-453.

14. Fitzgerald RH Jr, Nolan DR, Ilstrup DM, Van Scoy RE, Washington JA II, Coventry MB: Deep wound sepsis following total hip arthroplasty. *J Bone Joint Surg Am* 1977;59(7):847-855.

15. Hood RW, Insall JN: Infected total knee joint replacement arthroplasties, in Evarts CM, ed: *Surgery of the Musculoskeletal System.* New York, NY, Churchill Livingstone, 1983, vol 4, pp 173-195.

16. Karas SE, Gebhardt EM, Kenzora JE, Thornhill TS: Total hip arthroplasty for osteonecrosis following renal transplantation. *Orthop Trans* 1984;8:379-380.

17. Poss R, Thornhill TS, Ewald FC, Thomas WH, Batte NJ, Sledge CB: Factors influencing the incidence and outcome of infection following total joint arthroplasty. *Clin Orthop Relat Res* 1984;182:117-126.

18. Salvati EA, Robinson RP, Zeno SM, Koslin BL, Brause BD, Wilson PD Jr: Infection rates after 3175 total hip and total knee replacements performed with and without a horizontal unidirectional filtered air-flow system. *J Bone Joint Surg Am* 1982;64(4):525-535.

19. Thomas BJ, Moreland JR, Amstutz HC: Infection after total joint arthroplasty from distal extremity sepsis. *Clin Orthop Relat Res* 1983;181:121-125.

20. Wilson MG, Kelley K, Thornhill TS: Infection as a complication of total knee-replacement arthroplasty: Risk factors and treatment in sixty-seven cases. *J Bone Joint Surg Am* 1990;72(6):878-883.

21. Garner RW, Mowat AG, Hazleman BL: Wound healing after operations of patients with rheumatoid arthritis. *J Bone Joint Surg Br* 1973;55(1):134-144.

22. Thornhill TS, Maguire JH: Infected total knee arthroplasty, in Scott WN, ed: *Total Knee Revision Arthroplasty.* New York, NY, Grune & Stratton, 1987, pp 79-98.

23. Nelson CL: Prevention of sepsis. *Clin Orthop Relat Res* 1987;222:66-72.

24. Petty W, Bryan RS, Coventry MB, Peterson LF: Infection after total knee arthroplasty. *Orthop Clin North Am* 1975;6(4):1005-1014.

25. Menon TJ, Thjellesen D, Wroblewski BM: Charnley low-friction arthroplasty in diabetic patients. *J Bone Joint Surg Br* 1983;65(5):580-581.

26. Rayfield EJ, Ault MJ, Keusch GT, Brothers MJ, Nechemias C, Smith H: Infection and diabetes: The case for glucose control. *Am J Med* 1982;72(3):439-450.

27. Robertson HD, Polk HC Jr: The mechanism of infection in patients with diabetes mellitus: A review of leukocyte malfunction. *Surgery* 1974;75(1):123-128.

28. Galat DD, McGovern SC, Larson DR, Harrington JR, Hanssen AD, Clarke HD: Surgical treatment of early wound complications following primary total knee arthroplasty. *J Bone Joint Surg Am* 2009;91(1):48-54.

29. Greene KA, Wilde AH, Stulberg BN: Preoperative nutritional status of total joint patients: Relationship to postoperative wound complications. *J Arthroplasty* 1991;6(4):321-325.

30. Del Savio GC, Zelicof SB, Wexler LM, et al: Preoperative nutritional status and outcome of elective total hip replacement. *Clin Orthop Relat Res* 1996;326:153-161.

31. Parvizi J, Sullivan TA, Pagnano MW, Trousdale RT, Bolander ME: Total joint arthroplasty in human immunodeficiency virus-positive patients: An alarming rate of early failure. *J Arthroplasty* 2003;18(3):259-264.

32. Vilar-Compte D, Mohar A, Sandoval S, de la Rosa M, Gordillo P, Volkow P: Surgical site infections at the National Cancer Institute in Mexico: A case-control study. *Am J Infect Control* 2000;28(1):14-20.

33. Patel VP, Walsh M, Sehgal B, Preston C, DeWal H, Di Cesare PE: Factors associated with prolonged wound drainage after primary total hip and knee arthroplasty. *J Bone Joint Surg Am* 2007;89(1):33-38.

34. Lee GC, Pagnano MW, Hanssen AD: Total knee arthroplasty after prior bone or joint sepsis about the knee. *Clin Orthop Relat Res* 2002;404:226-231.

35. Strausbaugh LJ, Crossley KB, Nurse BA, Thrupp LD: Antimicrobial resistance in long-term-care facilities. *Infect Control Hosp Epidemiol* 1996;17(2):129-140.

36. Periti P, Mini E, Mosconi G: Antimicrobial prophylaxis in orthopaedic surgery: The role of teicoplanin. [Erratum appears in *J Antimicrob Chemother* 1998;42(6):840.] *J Antimicrob Chemother* 1998;41(3):329-340.

37. Page CP, Bohnen JM, Fletcher JR, McManus AT, Solomkin JS, Wittmann DH: Antimicrobial prophylaxis for surgical wounds: Guidelines for clinical care. *Arch Surg* 1993;128(1):79-88.

38. Mauerhan DR, Nelson CL, Smith DL, et al: Prophylaxis against infection in total joint arthroplasty: One day of cefuroxime compared with three days of cefazolin. *J Bone Joint Surg Am* 1994;76(1):39-45.

39. Patzakis MJ, Wilkins J, Kumar J, Holtom P, Greenbaum B, Ressler R: Comparison of the results of bacterial cultures from multiple sites in chronic osteomyelitis of long bones: A prospective study. *J Bone Joint Surg Am* 1994;76(5):664-666.

40. Gilbert DN, Moellering RC, Sande MA: *The Sanford Guide to Antimicrobial Therapy*, ed 35. Hyde Park, VT, 2005, p 125.

41. Dellinger EP, Gross PA, Barrett TL, et al: Quality standard for antimicrobial prophylaxis in surgical procedures. *Clin Infect Dis* 1994;18(3):422-427.

42. American Society of Health-System Pharmacists: ASHP therapeutic guidelines on antimicrobial prophylaxis in surgery. *Am J Health Syst Pharm* 1999;56(18):1839-1888.

43. Finkelstein R, Rabino G, Mashiah T, et al: Vancomycin versus cefazolin prophylaxis for cardiac surgery in the setting of a high prevalence of methicillin-resistant staphylococcal infections. *J Thorac Cardiovasc Surg* 2002;123(2):326-332.

44. Vuorisalo S, Pokela R, Syrjälä H: Comparison of vancomycin and cefuroxime for infection prophylaxis in coronary artery bypass surgery. *Infect Control Hosp Epidemiol* 1998;19(4):234-239.

45. Burke JF: The effective period of preventive antibiotic action in experimental incisions and dermal lesions. *Surgery* 1961;50:161-168.

46. Fukatsu K, Saito H, Matsuda T, Ikeda S, Furukawa S, Muto T: Influences of type and duration of antimicrobial prophylaxis on an outbreak of methicillin-resistant Staphylococcus aureus and on the incidence of wound infection. *Arch Surg* 1997;132(12):1320-1325.

47. Classen DC, Evans RS, Pestotnik SL, Horn SD, Menlove RL, Burke JP: The timing of prophylactic administration of antibiotics and the risk of surgical-wound infection. *N Engl J Med* 1992;326(5):281-286.

48. Auerbach AD: Prevention of surgical site infections, in Shojania KG, Duncan BW, McDonald KM, et al, eds: *Making Health Care Safer: A Critical Analysis of Patient Safety Practices.* Rockville, MD, Agency for Healthcare Research and Quality, 2001, pp 221-224.

49. American Academy of Orthopaedic Surgeons: Information statement. Recommendations for the use of intravenous antibiotic prophylaxis in primary total joint arthroplasty. Available at http://www.aaos.org/about/papers/advistmt/1027.asp. Accessed July 13, 2011.

50. Nelson CL, Green TG, Porter RA, Warren RD: One day versus seven days of preventive antibiotic therapy in orthopedic surgery. *Clin Orthop Relat Res* 1983;176:258-263.

51. Bethune DW, Blowers R, Parker M, Pask EA: Dispersal of staphylococcus aureus by patients and surgical staff. *Lancet* 1965;1(7383):480-483.

52. Ritter MA: Operating room environment. *Clin Orthop Relat Res* 1999;369:103-109.

53. Dalstrom DJ, Venkatarayappa I, Manternach AL, Palcic MS, Heyse BA, Prayson MJ: Time-dependent contamination of opened sterile operating-room trays. *J Bone Joint Surg Am* 2008;90(5):1022-1025.

54. Baird RA, Nickel FR, Thrupp LD, Rucker S, Hawkins B: Splash basin contamination in orthopaedic surgery. *Clin Orthop Relat Res* 1984;187:129-133.

55. Andersson BM, Lidgren L, Schalén C, Steen A: Contamination of irrigation solutions in an operating theatre. *Infect Control* 1984;5(7):339-341.

56. Strange-Vognsen HH, Klareskov B: Bacteriologic contamination of suction tips during hip arthroplasty. *Acta Orthop Scand* 1988;59(4):410-411.

57. Greenough CG: An investigation into contamination of operative suction. *J Bone Joint Surg Br* 1986;68(1):151-153.

58. Charnley J, Eftekhar N: Penetration of gown material by organisms from the surgeon's body. *Lancet* 1969;1(7587):172-173.

59. Blom A, Estela C, Bowker K, MacGowan A, Hardy JR: The passage of bacteria through surgical drapes. *Ann R Coll Surg Engl* 2000;82(6):405-407.

60. Johnston DH, Fairclough JA, Brown J, Morris R: Rate of bacterial recolonization of the skin after preparation: Four methods compared. *Br J Surg* 1987;74(1):64.

61. Fairclough JA, Johnson D, Mackie I: The prevention of wound contamination by skin organisms by the preoperative application of an iodophor impregnated plastic adhesive drape. *J Int Med Res* 1986;14(2):105-109.

62. Turner RS: Laminar air flow: Its original surgical application and long-term results. *J Bone Joint Surg Am* 1974;56(2):430-435.

63. Ritter MA, Olberding EM, Malinzak RA: Ultraviolet lighting during orthopaedic surgery and the rate of infection. *J Bone Joint Surg Am* 2007;89(9):1935-1940.

CHAPTER 6

MANAGEMENT OF BONE LOSS IN REVISION TOTAL KNEE ARTHROPLASTY

GORDON H. STOCK, MD
MATTHEW S. AUSTIN, MD
R. MICHAEL MENEGHINI, MD

INTRODUCTION

Primary total knee arthroplasty (TKA) is one of the most effective orthopaedic surgical procedures.[1,2] Most of these surgeries are successful in reducing pain and restoring function. A small percentage fail, however, and revision surgery is required. The leading causes of these failures are osteolysis due to polyethylene wear, loosening, instability, and infection.[3] The number of primary TKAs performed is expected to rise dramatically over the coming decades,[4,5] with an associated increase in the number of revision surgeries.[5,6] The goals of revision surgery are restoration of function through adequate fixation, proper ligament balancing, and restoration of the joint line. To meet these goals, the surgeon should anticipate and understand the bone loss associated with failed TKA as well as the treatment options for managing bone loss in the revision setting.

CLASSIFICATION OF BONE LOSS

The two most commonly used classification systems describing bone loss associated with TKA are the Anderson Orthopaedic Research Institute (AORI) bone defect classification[7] and the University of Pennsylvania (UPenn) system.[8] Both classification systems are useful and have been validated with respect to their ability to predict the bone loss that will be encountered intraoperatively based on preoperative radiographs.[9]

The AORI system has the advantage of ease of use and radiographic application. The UPenn classification is a useful research tool but is more cumbersome to apply. For these reasons, we use the AORI system more commonly in the clinical setting and the UPenn classification in the research setting.

Three types of bone defects are described in the AORI system. The type depends on the amount of metaphyseal bone remaining on the distal femur and proximal tibia (Table 1). In type 1 defects, small (< 1 cm) cancellous bone defects are present but the metaphyseal bone is intact. In type 2 defects, the metaphyseal cancellous and cortical bone is significantly damaged. Type 2 defects are further stratified into types 2A and 2B, depending on whether one or both condyles or plateaus are involved. Type 3 defects involve severe deficiency of the metaphyseal bone.

Dr. Austin or an immediate family member serves as a paid consultant to or is an employee of Zimmer and has received research or institutional support from DePuy. Dr. Meneghini or an immediate family member serves as a paid consultant to or is an employee of Stryker; has received research or institutional support from Stryker; and has received non-income support (such as equipment or services), commercially derived honoraria, or other non–research-related funding (such as paid travel) from Stryker. Neither Dr. Stock nor any immediate family member has received anything of value from or owns stock in a commercial company or institution related directly or indirectly to the subject of this chapter.

TABLE 1 Anderson Orthopaedic Research Institute (AORI) Bone Defect Classification

Defect Type	Description	Associated Bone Loss
Type 1 (F1/T1)	Metaphyseal rim intact Joint line intact Small defects (<1 cm)	
Type 2A (F2A/T2A)	Significant cancellous bone defect limited to one femoral condyle or one side of the tibial plateau Relatively intact metaphyseal bone	
Type 2B (F2B/T2B)	Significant cancellous bone defect involving both femoral condyles or both sides of the tibial plateau Relatively intact metaphyseal bone	
Type 3 (F3/T3)	Large metaphyseal rim defects with associated significant cancellous bone loss	

Treatment depends on the type of bone loss encountered (**Table 2**). Type 1 defects, which are limited to small areas (<1 cm) of cancellous bone loss at the level of the joint line on either of the distal femoral condyles or the proximal tibial plateau, are associated most commonly with revision procedures performed for aseptic loosening after primary TKA. The small size of these defects makes them amenable to treatment with knee components using standard augments,[10,11] allografts,[11-13] or cement.[11,14]

Type 2 and 3 defects are common in patients who have undergone previous revision surgeries. Often, a significant amount of cancellous bone is missing or damaged. When the loss is limited to one femoral condyle or one side of the tibial plateau, the defect is classified as type 2A. When the damage is more significant, involving both femoral condyles or the entire tibial plateau, then the defect is classified as a type 2B. Type 2 defects can be treated with morcellized allograft,[15] impaction grafting,[16-18] structural allograft,[19-23] contemporary modular revision systems that include metal augments,[10,24,25] metaphyseal sleeves, or porous metal cones.[25-29]

Type 3 defects, characterized by severe metaphyseal and uncontained bone loss, are more challenging. On the femoral side, the cancellous and cortical bone loss extends proximal to the level of the epicondyles. On the tibial side, the bone loss can extend distal to the tibial tubercle. The level of constraint needed at the time of reconstruction is dictated by the integrity of the ligaments. The management of type 3 defects can involve impaction grafting,[16,17,30,31] the use of contemporary revision systems with metaphyseal sleeves or porous metal cones,[25,27-29] structural allografts,[11,19-22,27-29,32] composite allografts,[33,34] or custom prostheses.[11]

The AORI classification is applied separately to the femur and the tibia. For example, a knee with an intact metaphyseal rim and 0.5 cm of localized cancellous bone loss on the tibia and large deficiencies of both distal femoral epicondyles would be classified as T1/F2B.

The classification system is applied during preoperative planning and serves to help anticipate the systems and/or implants that will be needed in the operating room. The knee is evaluated again intraoperatively, after the components have been removed and débridement has been completed. Encountering additional bone loss

TABLE 2	AORI Bone Loss Defects and Associated Treatment Options
AORI Defect	**Treatment Options**
Type 1	Cement alone
	Metal augments
	Morcellized allografts
Type 2	Cement in conjunction with other options
	Metal augments
	Morcellized allograft
	Impaction grafting
	Structural allograft
	Metaphyseal sleeves
	Porous metal cones
Type 3	Impaction grafting
	Structural allograft
	Metaphyseal sleeves
	Porous metal cones
	Composite allograft
	Custom prostheses

AORI = Anderson Orthopaedic Research Institute.

or ligament compromise is not unusual. This may necessitate a different treatment strategy, perhaps one that requires a higher level of constraint. The surgeon should anticipate this possibility before the surgery so that appropriate implants can be made available. This is particularly important in lower volume centers, where fewer reconstructive options may be routinely on hand.

PREOPERATIVE EVALUATION

The preoperative evaluation starts with the history and physical examination. The diagnosis is most commonly made by history, physical examination, and plain radiographs, but additional studies are occasionally needed to confirm the diagnosis and guide further treatment. For example, CT scans can be useful to determine malrotation of the femoral or tibial component.[35] All patients who are being considered for revision surgery should have an erythrocyte sedimentation rate (ESR) and C-reactive protein (CRP) level obtained preoperatively to screen for infection.[36]

FIGURE 1

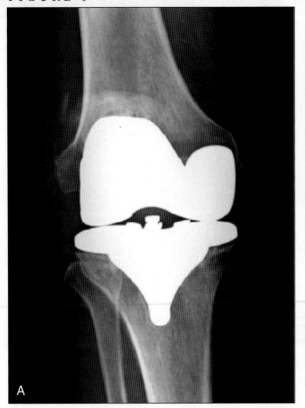
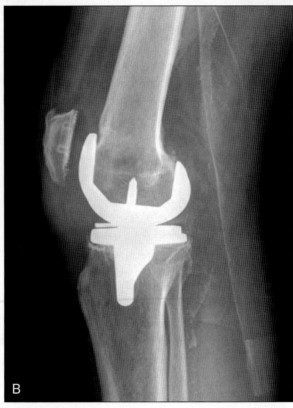

Preoperative AP (**A**) and lateral (**B**) radiographs of the knee of a patient with aseptic loosening that required revision. On the femoral side, both epicondyles appear to be intact. No defects are noted on the tibial side. On the basis of this preoperative radiographic information, the defect was classified as an AORI F1/T1 defect.

Good-quality radiographs are important in understanding both the qualitative and quantitative bone defects associated with revision arthroplasty. Weight-bearing AP, true lateral, and sunrise views of both knees should be obtained. Each radiograph is systematically evaluated. Using the AORI classification, the femur and the tibia are classified independently with respect to cancellous and cortical bone loss (**Figures 1** through **4**).

SURGICAL TECHNIQUE

Our preference is to use spinal anesthesia during revision cases. Preoperative antibiotics are given within 1 hour of making the incision. After appropriate positioning, the patient is prepared and draped, and previous skin inci-

sions are marked. When possible, previous incisions are incorporated to avoid necrosis of skin between incisions.

Adequate exposure is critical when performing revision TKA. There should be no hesitation to increase the length of the incision during the case to allow adequate exposure and visualization. With revision surgery, the soft-tissue planes are often blurred by extensive scar tissue. It is therefore important to extend the incision as necessary and work from normal tissue to re-create proper tissue planes.

The exposure starts with the skin incision. Dissection is carried down sharply to the level of the extensor mechanism. Small flaps are created both medially and laterally to facilitate closure; large subcutaneous flaps should be avoided. A medial parapatellar arthrotomy is

FIGURE 2

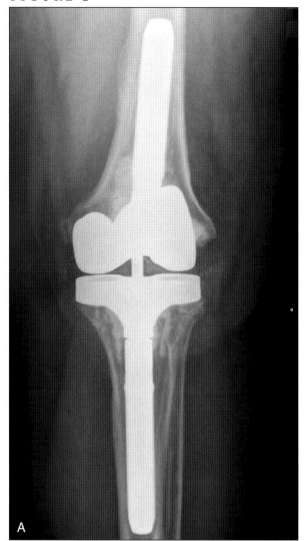
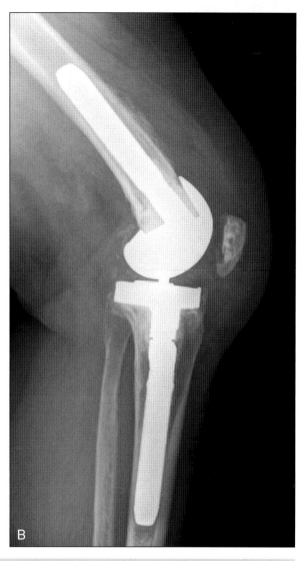

Preoperative AP (**A**) and lateral (**B**) radiographs of the knee of a patient with loosening of both the femoral and tibial components that required revision. The medial femoral condyle appears to be intact and to have no associated cancellous bone loss; however, only a shell of the lateral femoral condyle will remain after cement removal. On the tibial side, large cancellous defects will be present on both sides of the tibial plateau after component and cement removal. This was classified preoperatively as an AORI F2A/T2B defect.

performed, followed by a thorough intra-articular synovectomy to expose the implants and remaining bone stock and to re-create the lateral gutters.

After a medial release is performed, the knee is dislocated and the polyethylene insert is removed, if it is mod-

ular. Rather than everting the patella, it is subluxated to minimize tension on the extensor mechanism. If there is still extensive strain on the extensor mechanism when attempting to subluxate the patella, then a quadriceps snip can be performed. This will reduce the risk of traumatic

FIGURE 3

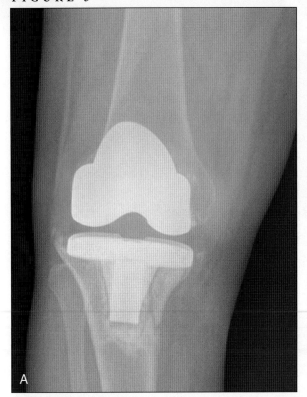 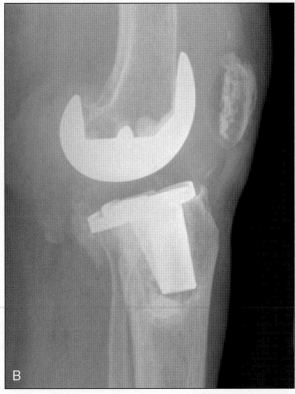

Preoperative AP (**A**) and lateral (**B**) radiographs of a knee that required revision demonstrate a periprosthetic fracture of the medial tibial plateau, radiolucency at the bone-cement interface, and subsidence of the tibial component. The femoral component appears well fixed. This was classified preoperatively as an AORI F1/T3 defect.

disruption of the extensor mechanism without adding additional restrictions in the postoperative period.[37] A careful posterior synovectomy is then completed.

Once the components are adequately exposed, the components are evaluated and implant removal is initiated as needed. The bone-cement or bone-implant interface is disrupted using a combination of osteotomes, an oscillating saw, and a ball-tipped burr. An explant device and slap hammer can then be used to remove the components. Care should be taken never to force or pry an implant loose. When removing the components, the amount of iatrogenic bone loss can be minimized by careful and methodical surgical technique.

Once the implants are removed, any cement is removed using osteotomes and the ball-tipped burr. The bony surfaces are then thoroughly débrided and the bone

is reevaluated using the AORI classification to categorize the bony defects. **Figures 5** through **8** are intraoperative views of the knees shown in **Figures 2** through **4.**

Each type of defect can be successfully treated with a unique array of options. **Table 2** lists these options, which are reviewed briefly below.

Cement

For AORI type 1 defects, cement alone is an excellent treatment option. Cement can be packed into small contained defects at the time of revision component placement. This has the advantage of being quick, inexpensive, and convenient. After the components are fully seated, excess cement is removed and discarded. Cementing of defects has the disadvantage of not restoring bone stock.

FIGURE 4

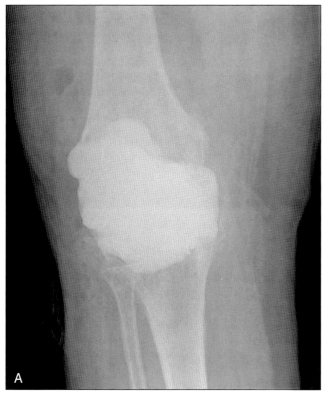 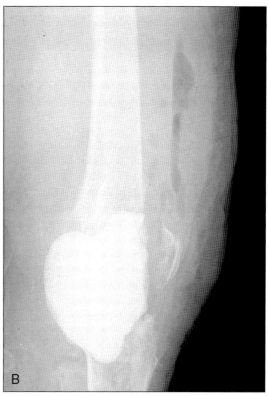

AP (**A**) and lateral (**B**) radiographs of the knee of a patient obtained after stage one of a two-stage revision for an infected total knee arthroplasty. Note the large metaphyseal defects on both the femur and the tibia. The AORI classification based on these radiographs and confirmed by intraoperative examination is F3/T3.

Cement is commonly used in conjunction with other treatment options for type 2 and type 3 defects. For example, when a type 3 defect is treated with a metaphyseal sleeve or porous metal cone and stemmed component, an area of bone loss between the remaining bone stock and the revision component commonly remains. In these instances, cement is often used as a filler material to provide some additional stability in the acute period, until osseointegration of the metaphyseal sleeve or porous metal cone is complete.

Metal Augments

Metal augments are typically used to treat AORI type 1 and type 2 defects. Contemporary revision systems all have modular metal augments that are available for use with the tibial and/or femoral component. Metal augments can effectively treat small peripheral cortical and cancellous bone defects. Biomechanically, a stronger construct is obtained when sloped peripheral defects are converted to a step-cut defect, which provides a horizontal and vertical surface for the augment to rest against.[10] These cuts are completed easily using instrumentation and an oscillating saw. The appropriately sized augment can then be selected and trialed. Metal augments have the advantage of being quick, convenient, and versatile. Augments of various sizes that can be positioned on the distal femur or posterior femoral condyles or under the tibial tray are readily available with contemporary revision systems. The position of the joint line can be manipulated when trialing components simply by changing the augment thickness. The actual augments to be implanted are then either

FIGURE 5

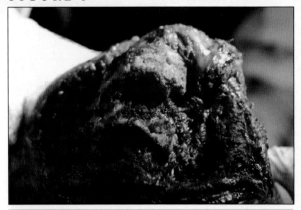

Intraoperative photograph of the same knee shown in Figure 1 after components have been removed and débridement completed. Small (< 1 cm) areas of bone loss are present. The intraoperative AORI classification is F1/T1, unchanged from the preoperative evaluation.

FIGURE 6

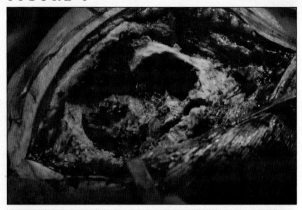

Intraoperative photograph of the same knee shown in Figure 2 after components and cement have been removed. The metaphyseal rim surrounding the tibial plateau is intact, but there is a significant loss of tibial cancellous bone, which also was noted on the preoperative radiographs. On the femoral side, the medial epicondyle is intact, but there is a fracture of the lateral epicondyle that was unappreciated on the preoperative radiographs, changing the classification of the femoral defect to type F3 rather than F2A as suspected on the preoperative evaluation. Therefore, the intraoperative classification is F3/T2B.

cemented or mechanically attached to the final implant before component implantation. Like cement, augments do not restore bone stock.

Morcellized Allograft

Unlike cement or metal augments, bone grafting has the advantage of restoring bone stock. This can be particularly important in younger patients in whom additional revision procedures are anticipated in the future.

Morcellized allograft can be used when treating AORI type 1 and type 2 defects in which the metaphyseal rim is intact. The primary advantage of using morcellized allograft is the potential to restore bone stock. As part of the débridement process, a burr is typically used to remove sclerotic bone down to an underlying bleeding cancellous bed. After thorough débridement is completed, allograft bone is placed within the contained defects before placement of the final components.

Impaction Grafting

Impaction grafting is most commonly used with AORI type 2 and type 3 defects. Similar to morcellized allograft, impaction grafting has the ability to reconstitute bone stock and is particularly attractive for the younger patient. Unlike augments, which often require additional removal of bone to obtain a step-cut configuration,

impaction grafting can be used with irregularly shaped defects. It is typically used for contained defects, but the addition of wire mesh to enclose metaphyseal defects has extended its application to uncontained defects.

One disadvantage of impaction grafting is the possibility of fracture or perforation of metaphyseal or diaphyseal bone while impacting the allograft. Another disadvantage of this technique is the time required to properly impact the allograft.

The surgical technique before impaction grafting is similar for all management options. The prosthesis is then trialed to determine the proper size and stem length of the implants. A trial stem that is several millimeters larger than the anticipated final stem is placed into the intramedullary canal. To avoid malalignment, this stem should be in the exact position required for the final components.

Morcellized bone graft is then progressively impacted in layers around the stem, continuing until the metaphysis has been filled. During impaction, there is a risk of fracture or perforation of the metaphyseal or diaphyseal

FIGURE 7

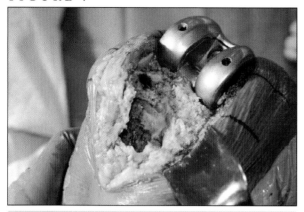

Intraoperative photograph shows an AORI type 3 tibial defect. Note the large anteromedial metaphyseal defect. This is the same defect shown in Figure 3.

FIGURE 8

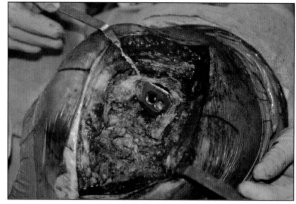

Intraoperative photograph shows a metaphyseal sleeve trial in place on the femur shown in Figure 6.

bone. The surgeon should be prepared to appropriately fix or bypass these iatrogenic fractures or perforations. Once the impaction process is complete, the trial stem is carefully removed. The final components are then cemented into place and excess cement is removed.

Structural Allograft

Another option to treat AORI type 2 and type 3 defects involves the use of structural, or bulk, allograft. Structural allograft is typically reserved for younger patients in whom the goal is to restore bone stock or for larger defects that exceed the size of available metal augments associated with a revision system.

After débridement is completed, the metaphyseal bone is hemispherically reamed. Care must be taken not to create an uncontained defect by unintentionally reaming through the thin metaphyseal cortical bone. Once the recipient bed is prepared, the femoral head allograft is then prepared on the back table using a female reamer. The allograft is usually reamed to one size larger than the male reamer used to prepare the metaphyseal bone. A pulsatile lavage system can be used to irrigate and remove the marrow elements from the allograft head. The allograft is then impacted into place and provisionally held with Kirschner wires (K-wires). An oscillating saw is used to remove excess graft. A reamer or high-speed burr is used to reestablish communication with the intra-

medullary canal. Components are then trialed and adjustment made as necessary. Once the final components are in place, the K-wires are removed.

Metaphyseal Sleeves

Metaphyseal sleeves are commonly used to treat AORI type 2 and type 3 defects. The sleeves have the advantage that initial stability can be obtained at the time of the revision procedure and biologic final fixation.

After débridement is completed, the intramedullary canals are reamed. A conical reamer is introduced to prepare the metaphyseal bone for the smallest broach. Sequentially larger broaches are then used until the broach is stable axially and rotationally. These metaphyseal broaches serve as a trial sleeve and allow for stable trialing of the components. The final broach is slightly smaller than the final sleeve implant, to allow for press-fit fixation. Either posterior stabilized or hinged components can be used with the sleeves, depending on the degree of constraint required. **Figure 8** shows a metaphyseal sleeve trial in place on the same femur shown in Figure 6.

When impacting the broach longitudinally, it is critical that the joint line be reestablished in the proper position to facilitate gap balancing in flexion and extension. The meniscal scar can be a helpful landmark. Additionally, the medial and lateral epicondyles can be used as a reference to reestablish the proper joint line. The

FIGURE 9

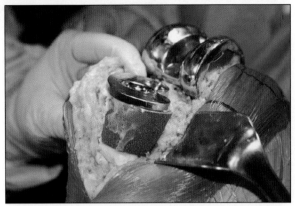

Intraoperative photograph shows a step-cut porous metal cone used to treat an AORI type 3 tibial defect. This is the same defect shown in Figures 3 and 7.

FIGURE 10

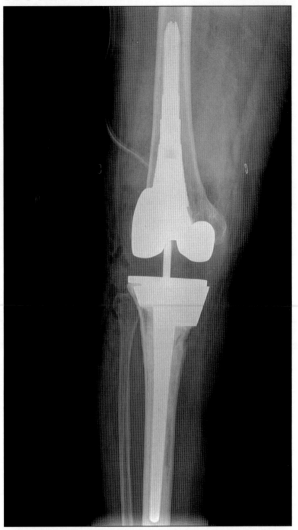

Postoperative AP radiograph of the patient shown in Figures 3, 7, and 9. This is an AORI type F1/T3 defect.

mean distance from the epicondyle to the joint line is 3.2 cm medially and 2.5 cm laterally. The transepicondylar axis can also be used to determine proper rotation of the femoral component.[38]

After the final femoral trials have been loosely assembled, the components are placed and the correct femoral and tibial rotation with respect to the sleeve orientation is established. The components are removed and the Morse taper between the sleeve and the distal femur or tibial tray is impacted. Components are then impacted into place. No cement is used on the metaphyseal sleeve, but cement can be used on the femoral condyles or tibial tray to fill any remaining voids behind the components and to reestablish the shape of the metaphyseal bone. This minimizes irritation on the soft-tissue envelope and provides additional stability until osseointegration of the metaphyseal sleeve is complete.

Metaphyseal sleeves have the advantage of obtaining secure initial fixation in large defects. Additionally, there is not the concern of graft reabsorption associated with impaction grafting and bulk allograft techniques. Patients are typically allowed to be fully weight bearing immediately postoperatively.

Disadvantages of the sleeves include their cost and the potential for fracture when impacting the broach into deficient bone. Occasionally, when there is a heightened concern for fracture because of poor bone quality, a prophylactic cable can be placed to minimize the chance of creating or propagating an iatrogenic fracture. Sleeves also do not restore bone stock, and they may in fact require additional bone removal for implantation.

Porous Metal Cones

Porous metal cones are an alternative reconstruction technique used in AORI type 2 and type 3 defects. Like the porous sleeves, they have the advantage of creating a stable platform on which the revision components can be placed, allowing the patient to bear weight immediately postoperatively. They are impacted to obtain stability acutely using an interference fit between the bone and the porous cone implant. Long-term fixation is obtained through osseointegration. Cones are available in a wide variety of shapes and sizes that allow their use with both contained and uncontained defects. As with metaphyseal sleeves, the use of cones avoids concerns about graft resorption. The disadvantages of porous metal cones include their cost and the lack of bone stock reconstitution.

Surgical technique involves using a ream/broach system or a high-speed burr to mill the bone to maximize the contact between the remaining bone stock and the porous cone implant. The cone is then impacted into place. Typically, crushed allograft is packed into any voids that remain between the implant and the cancellous or cortical bone against which it is impacted. Once the porous metal cone is in place, a stemmed component (either cemented or uncemented) can then be placed through the cone. We often use an uncemented stem but cement the component proximally in the metaphysis at the level of the porous metal implant; the cement interdigitates nicely with the interior surface of the porous metal. It is important to note that the rotation of the tibial component is not dependent upon the rotational orientation of the porous metal implant. An example of a step-cut porous metal cone with the tibial component cemented in place is shown in **Figure 9**. This is the same AORI type 3 tibial defect shown in Figures 3 and 7.

Composite Allograft and Custom Prostheses

Composite allograft and custom prostheses are used infrequently now because advancements have been made in contemporary revision systems and the other treatment options outlined above for severe femoral or tibial bone loss. The use of composite allograft and custom prostheses is now limited to salvage cases in which other options are not feasible. Disadvantages include increased complications, including infection, nonunion, and fracture.[34]

Combined Techniques

In many instances, multiple techniques will be used in a single patient. For example, **Figure 10** is a postoper-

ative radiograph of a knee with an AORI type F1/T3 defect (the same knee shown in Figures 3, 7, and 9). On the femoral side, an uncemented stem was combined with a metaphyseal sleeve to obtain stable fixation. Distally, cement was used sparingly to fill the space between the backside of the femoral articulation and the sleeve. On the tibial side, there was a large, uncontained metaphyseal defect. A step-cut porous metal sleeve was used to obtain fixation in the proximal tibia and to serve as a platform on which the remainder of the tibial construct would sit. A cemented tibial component and stem were used.

POSTOPERATIVE MANAGEMENT

Postoperative management is tailored to the individual patient and is highly variable based on the degree of bone loss encountered, the reconstruction technique used, extensor mechanism compromise, soft-tissue quality, intraoperative findings, and the quality of initial fixation obtained in the operating room. With large allograft techniques, weight bearing is restricted until graft incorporation has occurred. This same restriction generally does not apply when cement, metal augments, porous sleeves, or cones are used.

COMPLICATIONS

Complications of revision TKA include failures from osteolysis due to polyethylene wear, loosening, instability, and infection. Revision TKA is associated with a higher complication rate than primary TKA.[39] This is particularly true for revision TKA in the younger patient (<60 years of age).[40]

Revision TKA is also associated with complications that are not typically encountered with primary TKA. For example, many revision procedures use stemmed components that can lead to end-of-stem pain,[41] and graft resorption may occur, leading to failure of the reconstruction.

Furthermore, there are complications that are technique-dependent. As discussed above, when using augments, a step-cut is more stable biomechanically and less prone to failure than a wedge-shaped augment used for an oblique defect.[10] With impaction grafting and structural allograft, there is a concern for graft reabsorption. Although complications cannot be eliminated altogether, an understanding of the principles associated with each technique can minimize such complications.

CONCLUSIONS

Bone loss associated with revision TKA will continue to pose a challenge to the reconstructive surgeon. The surgeon should understand the different types of bone loss and available surgical techniques appropriate for each defect to maximize the success of the procedure.

REFERENCES

1. Buechel FF Sr: Long-term followup after mobile-bearing total knee replacement. *Clin Orthop Relat Res* 2002;404:40-50.

2. Khaw FM, Kirk LM, Morris RW, Gregg PJ: A randomised, controlled trial of cemented versus cementless press-fit condylar total knee replacement: Ten-year survival analysis. *J Bone Joint Surg Br* 2002;84(5):658-666.

3. Sharkey PF, Hozack WJ, Rothman RH, Shastri S, Jacoby SM: Insall Award paper: Why are total knee arthroplasties failing today? *Clin Orthop Relat Res* 2002;404:7-13.

4. Kurtz S, Ong K, Lau E, Mowat F, Halpern M: Projections of primary and revision hip and knee arthroplasty in the United States from 2005 to 2030. *J Bone Joint Surg Am* 2007;89(4):780-785.

5. Kurtz SM, Lau E, Ong K, Zhao K, Kelly M, Bozic KJ: Future young patient demand for primary and revision joint replacement: National projections from 2010 to 2030. *Clin Orthop Relat Res* 2009;467(10):2606-2612.

6. Kurtz S, Mowat F, Ong K, Chan N, Lau E, Halpern M: Prevalence of primary and revision total hip and knee arthroplasty in the United States from 1990 through 2002. *J Bone Joint Surg Am* 2005;87(7):1487-1497.

7. Engh GA, Ammeen DJ: Bone loss with revision total knee arthroplasty: Defect classification and alternatives for reconstruction. *Instr Course Lect* 1999;48:167-175.

8. Nelson CL, Lonner JH, Rand JA, Lotke PA: Strategies of stem fixation and the role of supplemental bone graft in revision total knee arthroplasty. *J Bone Joint Surg Am* 2003;85(Suppl 1):S52-S57.

9. Mulhall KJ, Ghomrawi HM, Engh GA, Clark CR, Lotke P, Saleh KJ: Radiographic prediction of intraoperative bone loss in knee arthroplasty revision. *Clin Orthop Relat Res* 2006;446:51-58.

10. Chen F, Krackow KA: Management of tibial defects in total knee arthroplasty: A biomechanical study. *Clin Orthop Relat Res* 1994;305:249-257.

11. Gross AE: Revision total knee arthroplasty of bone grafts versus implant supplementation. *Orthopedics* 1997;20(9):843-844.

12. Toms AD, Barker RL, Jones RS, Kuiper JH: Impaction bone-grafting in revision joint replacement surgery. *J Bone Joint Surg Am* 2004;86(9):2050-2060.

13. Whiteside LA, Bicalho PS: Radiologic and histologic analysis of morselized allograft in revision total knee replacement. *Clin Orthop Relat Res* 1998;357:149-156.

14. Ritter MA, Harty LD: Medial screws and cement: A possible mechanical augmentation in total knee arthroplasty. *J Arthroplasty* 2004;19(5):587-589.

15. Benjamin J, Engh G, Parsley B, Donaldson T, Coon T: Morselized bone grafting of defects in revision total knee arthroplasty. *Clin Orthop Relat Res* 2001;392:62-67.

16. Bradley GW: Revision total knee arthroplasty by impaction bone grafting. *Clin Orthop Relat Res* 2000;371:113-118.

17. Lotke PA, Carolan GF, Puri N: Impaction grafting for bone defects in revision total knee arthroplasty. *Clin Orthop Relat Res* 2006;446:99-103.

18. Ries MD: Impacted cancellous autograft for contained bone defects in total knee arthroplasty. *Am J Knee Surg* 1996;9(2):51-54.

19. Clatworthy MG, Ballance J, Brick GW, Chandler HP, Gross AE: The use of structural allograft for uncontained defects in revision total knee arthroplasty: A minimum five-year review. *J Bone Joint Surg Am* 2001;83-A(3):404-411.

20. Engh GA, Ammeen DJ: Use of structural allograft in revision total knee arthroplasty in knees with severe tibial bone loss. *J Bone Joint Surg Am* 2007;89(12):2640-2647.

21. Ghazavi MT, Stockley I, Yee G, Davis A, Gross AE: Reconstruction of massive bone defects with allograft in revision total knee arthroplasty. *J Bone Joint Surg Am* 1997;79(1):17-25.

22. Mow CS, Wiedel JD: Structural allografting in revision total knee arthroplasty. *J Arthroplasty* 1996;11(3):235-241.

23. Stockley I, McAuley JP, Gross AE: Allograft reconstruction in total knee arthroplasty. *J Bone Joint Surg Br* 1992;74(3):393-397.

24. Patel JV, Masonis JL, Guerin J, Bourne RB, Rorabeck CH: The fate of augments to treat type-2 bone defects in revision knee arthroplasty. *J Bone Joint Surg Br* 2004;86(2):195-199.

25. Radnay CS, Scuderi GR: Management of bone loss: Augments, cones, offset stems. *Clin Orthop Relat Res* 2006;446:83-92.

26. Bobyn JD, Poggie RA, Krygier JJ, et al: Clinical validation of a structural porous tantalum biomaterial for adult reconstruction. *J Bone Joint Surg Am* 2004;86-A(Suppl 2):123-129.

27. Long WJ, Scuderi GR: Porous tantalum cones for large metaphyseal tibial defects in revision total knee arthroplasty: A minimum 2-year follow-up. *J Arthroplasty* 2009;24(7):1086-1092.

28. Meneghini RM, Lewallen DG, Hanssen AD: Use of porous tantalum metaphyseal cones for severe tibial bone loss during revision total knee replacement. *J Bone Joint Surg Am* 2008;90(1):78-84.

29. Meneghini RM, Lewallen DG, Hanssen AD: Use of porous tantalum metaphyseal cones for severe tibial bone loss during revision total knee replacement: Surgical technique. *J Bone Joint Surg Am* 2009;91(Suppl 2 Pt 1):131-138.

30. Lonner JH, Lotke PA, Kim J, Nelson C: Impaction grafting and wire mesh for uncontained defects in revision knee arthroplasty. *Clin Orthop Relat Res* 2002;404:145-151.

31. Suárez-Suárez MA, Murcia A, Maestro A: Filling of segmental bone defects in revision knee arthroplasty using morsellized bone grafts contained within a metal mesh. *Acta Orthop Belg* 2002;68(2):163-167.

32. Tsahakis PJ, Beaver WB, Brick GW: Technique and results of allograft reconstruction in revision total knee arthroplasty. *Clin Orthop Relat Res* 1994;303:86-94.

33. Harris AI, Poddar S, Gitelis S, Sheinkop MB, Rosenberg AG: Arthroplasty with a composite of an allograft and a prosthesis for knees with severe deficiency of bone. *J Bone Joint Surg Am* 1995;77(3):373-386.

34. Mnaymneh W, Emerson RH, Borja F, Head WC, Malinin TI: Massive allografts in salvage revisions of failed total knee arthroplasties. *Clin Orthop Relat Res* 1990;260:144-153.

35. Nicoll D, Rowley DI: Internal rotational error of the tibial component is a major cause of pain after total knee replacement. *J Bone Joint Surg Br* 2010;92(9):1238-1244.

36. Ghanem E, Parvizi J, Burnett RS, et al: Cell count and differential of aspirated fluid in the diagnosis of infection at the site of total knee arthroplasty. *J Bone Joint Surg Am* 2008;90(8):1637-1643.

37. Della Valle CJ, Berger RA, Rosenberg AG: Surgical exposures in revision total knee arthroplasty. *Clin Orthop Relat Res* 2006;446:59-68.

38. Stiehl JB, Abbott BD: Morphology of the transepicondylar axis and its application in primary and revision total knee arthroplasty. *J Arthroplasty* 1995;10(6):785-789.

39. Ong KL, Lau E, Suggs J, Kurtz SM, Manley MT: Risk of subsequent revision after primary and revision total joint arthroplasty. *Clin Orthop Relat Res* 2010;468(11):3070-3076.

40. Gioe TJ, Killeen KK, Grimm K, Mehle S, Scheltema K: Why are total knee replacements revised? Analysis of early revision in a community knee implant registry. *Clin Orthop Relat Res* 2004;428:100-106.

41. Barrack RL, Rorabeck C, Burt M, Sawhney J: Pain at the end of the stem after revision total knee arthroplasty. *Clin Orthop Relat Res* 1999;367:216-225.

MANAGEMENT OF EXTENSOR MECHANISM DISRUPTION AFTER TOTAL KNEE ARTHROPLASTY

FABIO OROZCO, MD
ALVIN ONG, MD

INTRODUCTION

Extensor mechanism disruption from quadriceps tendon rupture, patellar tendon rupture, or patellar fracture is an uncommon complication after total knee arthroplasty (TKA), with a reported incidence of 0.17% to 2.5%.[1-3] With advances in technology and surgical technique, more active and younger patients are undergoing TKA, so the incidence of extensor mechanism disruption is likely to increase. The surgical treatment options for the repair of disrupted extensor mechanisms include primary repair, autologous tissue augmentation, and allograft tissue reconstruction. Recent advances in the use of augmentation techniques for reconstruction have yielded promising results. Extensor mechanism disruptions can be differentiated into proximal extensor mechanism ruptures (quadriceps tendon) and distal extensor mechanism ruptures (patellar tendon). Periprosthetic patellar fractures following TKA occur infrequently; the reported incidence ranges from 0.2% to 21%.[4,5] Patellar fractures can also occur without resurfacing of the patella, but they are more prevalent if the patella has been resurfaced.[5] Asymptomatic nondisplaced patellar fractures can be treated nonsurgically. Surgical management is reserved for symptomatic patients with functional impairment.

ETIOLOGY

Extensor Mechanism Rupture

The etiology of extensor mechanism disruption is multifactorial. Risk factors include trauma, patient comorbidities, prior knee surgery, anatomic constraints, surgical technique, and prosthetic design. Patient comorbidities include obesity, steroid use, Parkinson disease, diabetes mellitus, rheumatoid arthritis, systemic lupus erythematosus, and chronic renal failure.

Extensor mechanism rupture can also be associated with particular surgical techniques, such as a lateral release or quadriceps snip. Other risk factors include multiple previous operations, difficult exposure in arthrofibrotic and/or revision cases, extensive release of the patellar tendon at the time of surgical exposure, manipulation of a stiff knee, and prior distal realignment procedures for patellar maltracking.

Dr. Orozco or an immediate family member serves as a paid consultant to or is an employee of Stryker, has received research or institutional support from Pfizer and AkPharma, and has received nonincome support (such as equipment or services), commercially derived honoraria, or other non–research-related funding (such as paid travel) from Pfizer. Dr. Ong or an immediate family member is a member of a speakers' bureau or has made paid presentations on behalf of Pfizer, serves as a paid consultant to or is an employee of Stryker, and has received research or institutional support from Pfizer and AkPharma.

Patellar Fracture

The etiologies of patellar fractures include trauma, implant malalignment, obesity, overresection of bone, high activity level, and increased range of motion. The blood supply to the patella can be compromised intraoperatively, during lateral retinacular release or resection of the fat pad or from aggressive stripping of soft tissue around the patellar bone or heat necrosis from the saw blade. A compromised blood supply can lead to osteonecrosis and subsequent fracture of the patella.

CLASSIFICATION
Extensor Mechanism Rupture

No useful accepted classification system exists for extensor mechanism disruption after TKA. Extensor mechanism ruptures can be categorized by location (either proximal [quadriceps tear] or distal [patellar tendon tear]) and then subclassified according to whether the tear occurs in the midsubstance or at the distal or proximal insertion. Alternatively, they can be graded as acute (<2 weeks) or chronic (>2 weeks). Finally, ruptures can be qualified as partial-thickness or full-thickness tears, depending on the presence or absence of active extension of the knee and MRI findings.

Periprosthetic Patellar Fracture

The most widely accepted classification system for periprosthetic patellar fractures after TKA is the Mayo Clinic classification, which offers guidance for optimal treatment.[5] In this classification system, patellar fractures are categorized by the stability of the patellar implant and the integrity of the extensor mechanism. In this classification system, fractures are divided into three types according to the stability of the patellar implant and the status of the extensor mechanism, with the third type further divided into two subtypes depending on bone quality (**Table 1**).

CLINICAL FINDINGS
Extensor Mechanism Rupture
Quadriceps Tendon Rupture

Patients with quadriceps tendon rupture usually have a history of a fall or a vigorous contraction of the thigh. They present with severe pain, weakness, and ambulatory dysfunction. Pain is localized just above the patella. Physical examination findings include swelling of the

TABLE 1 Mayo Clinic Classification of Periprosthetic Patellar Fractures

Fracture Type	Characteristics	
	Patellar Implant	Extensor Mechanism
I	Stable	Intact
II	Stable	Disrupted
IIIa (good bone stock)	Loose	Intact
IIIb (poor bone stock[a])	Loose	Intact

[a]Poor bone stock is defined as bone <10 mm thick or with marked comminution.

knee with tenderness in the quadriceps tendon. A very important and common clinical finding is a palpable defect above the superior pole of the patella. The patient will also have weak or no active extension of the knee.

Patellar Tendon Rupture

Patients with patellar tendon rupture may or may not report a history of injury. The patient reports ambulatory dysfunction and pain at the region just below the patella or at the tibial tubercle. On physical examination, there is swelling and a high-riding patella. The patient has weak or no active extension of the knee.

Periprosthetic Patellar Fracture

Patients with periprosthetic patellar fractures present with knee effusion, anterior knee pain, and ambulatory dysfunction. Most patients report discomfort or difficulty rising from a seated position or ascending or descending stairs. A history of injury, such as a fall or direct impact to the anterior knee, is common. Physical examination reveals tenderness over the patella. With a displaced fracture, a defect or crepitus may be palpable. In type II fractures, appreciable extensor weakness or extensor lag is often noted. Flexion is usually not affected except in a patient with a history of acute injury with associated tense effusion or hemarthrosis.

IMAGING
Extensor Mechanism Rupture

AP, lateral, and sunrise views of the knee should be obtained. It is helpful to compare these radiographs with those taken immediately after the TKA. With a quadriceps tendon rupture, patella infera may be seen on the lateral view, and the sunrise view will usually show excessive tilt of the patella. With a complete patellar tendon rupture, on the other hand, patella alta is the most common radiographic finding on the lateral view. Bony fragments may be seen superior or inferior to the patella at or near the tibial tubercle, indicating avulsion of the tendon.

Clinical correlation is indicated in patients with normal radiographs and positive findings on examination; normal radiographs do not rule out tendon injury or rupture. MRI of the knee may be necessary when the diagnosis cannot be made with clinical and radiographic examination. MRI can also be helpful to differentiate between partial- and full-thickness ruptures.

Periprosthetic Patellar Fractures

AP, lateral, and sunrise views must be obtained in the setting of anterior pain after a fall. The lateral and sunrise views are especially helpful in the diagnosis and assessment of patellar fracture. The AP view is less helpful because the femoral implant typically obscures the patella. Other imaging studies, such as CT and MRI, have little value in the management of patellar fractures.

TREATMENT
Extensor Mechanism Rupture
Quadriceps Tendon Rupture

Partial tears of the quadriceps may be treated nonsurgically, but complete tendon ruptures require surgical treatment. Dobbs et al[6] reported on 34 patients who had ruptures of the quadriceps tendon postoperatively; 11 had complete tears, and the remaining 23 had partial tears. Seven patients with partial tears and one patient with a complete tear were treated nonsurgically. Nonsurgical treatment led to a satisfactory outcome in all patients in the partial quadriceps rupture group. Nonsurgical treatment consisted of immobilization of the knee in extension for 6 weeks and crutch ambulation for 6 weeks. This was followed by gentle range of motion. Only one patient had a residual 10° extensor lag; the other six patients had full active extension of the knee with no recurrence of quadriceps rupture. In contrast, nonsurgical treatment led to poor results in the patient with a complete quadriceps tear. At 1-year follow-up, this patient had no active knee extension and had a 3-cm palpable defect at the site of the quadriceps tendon. The authors concluded that nonsurgical treatment is not recommended in patients with complete rupture of the tendon.

Patellar Tendon Rupture

Patellar tendon ruptures after TKA are difficult to treat. The blood supply and tissue quality of the tendon may be compromised. Exposure may have been difficult, and the tendon may have been partially or completely avulsed from the tibial tubercle, especially during revision surgery.

Attempts at primary repair following a TKA rarely restore extensor function,[2] and postoperative ruptures of the patellar tendon require autograft or allograft reconstruction.[7-9] Graft options include semitendinosus autograft, medial gastrocnemius flap, Achilles tendon allograft, and whole extensor mechanism allograft. The most common allograft of choice is an Achilles tendon allograft. Achilles graft with intact calcaneus bone is preferred. The calcaneus bone is recessed into a prepared bed in the tibial tubercle. The Achilles tendon acts as a new patellar tendon and is sutured to the native extensor mechanism with nonabsorbable suture. Rand et al[3] reported on patellar tendon ruptures in 18 knees in 17 patients. Treatment consisted of observation in two cases, suture repair in nine knees, staple fixation in four, xenograft reconstruction in two, and semitendinosus reconstruction in one. Results were consistently poor in all patients treated with observation and primary suture repair. The only treatment techniques that resulted in successful outcomes were staple fixation, which was successful in two of four knees, and the bovine xenograft reconstruction, which was successful in both of the knees in which it was used. The authors concluded that patellar tendon rupture in TKA should not be treated with observation or primary repair alone. Unfortunately, surgical treatment results were variable and carried a high complication rate. Cadambi and Engh[1] reported on seven patients in whom autologous semitendinosus graft was used to reconstruct the patellar tendon. In their technique, the harvested semitendinosus tendon was routed into the distal patellar bone or quadriceps tendon and sutured to itself and to the retinaculum on the proximal tibia. They achieved good success with this technique, reporting a mean extensor lag of 10° in their seven patients at a mean of 30 months. Jaureguito et al[10] used medial gastrocnemius muscle flaps to reconstruct the ruptured patellar tendon in six patients. In their technique, the medial gastrocnemius was split from its attachment to the Achilles tendon and then mobilized and sutured to the retinaculum and remaining patellar tendon. At a mean follow-up of 26 months, mean range of motion was 100° and the mean extensor lag was 24°. Two complications were reported in their series; both were related to stiffness. The authors concluded that the medial gastrocnemius flap is a reliable option in the treatment of patellar tendon rupture in TKA. Emerson et al[11] used whole extensor mechanism allograft with a cemented patellar prosthesis in nine patients. At a mean follow-up of 4.1 years (range, 2.3 to 7.0 years), six patients had full active extension, and three had extensor lag ranging from 20° to 40°. Allografts at the tibial attachment site healed successfully in all patients. Two complications occurred—one failure of graft incorporation at the quadriceps attachment junction, and another at the patella–patellar tendon junction. One patient fractured the allograft patella during a severe fall. The authors reported mixed results and warned that the long-term durability of this technique is not known. Crossett et al[8] reported on the use of fresh-frozen Achilles tendon allograft in the reconstruction of patellar tendon rupture. In their series of nine patients, the patellar tendon ruptured in five patients following primary TKA and in four patients following revision TKA. The technique the authors used is very similar to the extensor mechanism reconstruction with Achilles tendon allograft described below under Selected Surgical Techniques: Avulsion From the Tibial Tubercle. The mean extensor lag after reconstruction was 3°, and mean flexion was 107°. Two graft failures occurred; they were successfully repaired. Although the patella migrated proximally an average of 18 mm, the authors reported no effect on extensor function. They concluded that the use of Achilles tendon allograft is reliable in the reconstruction of patellar tendon ruptures following TKA. Burnett et al[9] recommended that the allograft tendon be initially tensioned tight in extension to prevent extensor lag postoperatively.

Patellar Fracture
Type I Fractures
Type I fractures, defined as fractures in which the patellar implant is stable and the extensor mechanism is intact, are best treated nonsurgically. These fractures are frequently asymptomatic, and patients present with no functional limitations. Most are diagnosed on routine follow-up radiographs. Asymptomatic patients can be treated with observation. Patients who have swelling and pain can be treated with 4 to 6 weeks of immobilization followed by resumption of activities as tolerated. Ortiguera and Berry[5] reported that 37 of 38 patients with type I fractures (82%) had no pain or extensor mechanism instability or weakness at last follow-up. Only one patient with late failure required surgical intervention. In the rare cases in which surgery becomes necessary in a type I fracture, treatment involves excision of a marginal fragment/nonunion with soft-tissue repair of the extensor mechanism to the remaining patella.

Type II Fractures
Type II fractures are defined as patellar fractures associated with disruption of the extensor mechanism. The patellar implant remains well fixed. The patient usually reports a fall or injury. Physical examination findings include full or partial loss of active extension with associated swelling and pain. Radiographs typically reveal polar fractures of the patella at the superior or inferior periphery of the patella. Most of the patellar mass is usually preserved. Type II fractures are uncommon. In the Ortiguera and Berry[5] study of patellar fractures, only 12 (15%) were type II fractures. Most type II fractures require open reduction and internal fixation or suture repair. Fixation can consist of screw or wire fixation if the polar fragment is significant in size. If the polar fracture fragment is too small to receive fixation hardware, excision of the fragment (partial patellectomy) can be performed, with advancement of the tendon onto bone. After the polar fragment has been excised, tendon advancement can be performed. In the Ortiguera and Berry series,[5] 6 of 12 type II fractures were treated with open reduction and internal fixation, and 5 of 12 fractures were treated with partial patellectomy and tendon advancement. The authors reported a 50% complication rate. Of the 12 knees, 5 required reoperation and 7 had pain or patellar/extensor mechanism instability or weakness. Resolution of pain and the return to full functional capacity was seen in only 50% of the patients. Most reported some pain and functional limitation at last follow-up.

Type III Fractures

Type III fractures are defined as patellar fractures associated with a loose patellar implant. Type III fractures are subdivided into those with good bone stock (type IIIa) and those with poor bone stock (type IIIb). Poor bone stock is defined as a patellar bone thickness less than 10 mm or severe comminution that rules out internal fixation or another resurfacing procedure. Ortiguera and Berry[5] reported on 28 type III patellar fractures. Of the 28, 12 had reasonable bone stock (type IIIa); 4 of these were treated with observation, and the other 8 were treated surgically. Of the 8 treated surgically, 5 were treated with patellar component resection and internal fixation of the fracture. An unacceptable number of complications and reoperations occurred in the surgically managed group. Of the 4 patients treated with observation, 2 remained symptomatic at latest follow-up.

Of the 28 type III fractures in the series of Ortiguera and Berry,[5] 16 had poor bone stock (type IIIb); 4 of these were treated with observation, and 12 were treated surgically. Only one of four knees treated nonsurgically had pain at latest follow-up. Of the 12 surgically managed knees, 7 had pain and patellar instability or weakness at latest follow-up. Ortiguera and Berry[5] recommend that type IIIa patellar fractures be managed with revision of the patellar component or resection of the patellar component with patelloplasty. For type IIIb fractures, they recommend removal of the patellar implant with partial or complete patellectomy.

Porous tantalum patellar components have been developed recently for the treatment of substantial patellar bone loss.[12] Although this technique was described for marked bone loss and not necessarily for patellar fractures, it offers a viable alternative to partial or complete patellectomy for type IIIb patellar fractures in which the bone stock prevents the use of a standard patellar component. In our experience with 11 patients with type IIIb fractures that were treated with a porous tantalum patellar component, most patients (9 of 11) reported pain relief, resolution of effusion, and improved functional ability (Hoke D, Orozco F, Ong A: Trabecular metal augmentation component for patella fracture. Poster presentation at TribOS Articulating Science Meeting. Noosa, Queensland, Australia, Sept 2008).

FIGURE 1

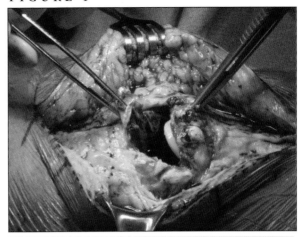

Full-thickness medial and lateral flaps are elevated for exposure of the knee for extensor mechanism repair.

Two failures were seen at latest follow-up. The first failure was due to superior pole fracture of the remnant patellar shell. These polar fractures occur because of fatigue failure due to weakness of the thin cortical shell seen in these patients, as well as the stress riser created by the edge of the metal shell on the compromised bone. The second failure was due to nonhealing or failure of ingrowth of the trabecular implant into the bone. This technique requires adequate blood supply for healing to occur and therefore is highly patient dependent.

PREOPERATIVE PREPARATION AND SURGICAL APPROACH

The leg should be prepared and draped with the same technique used for a primary TKA, with the same considerations for anesthesia. The procedure is done under tourniquet control to improve visualization. The use of preoperative antibiotics is recommended. The knee is approached through the preexisting surgical scar. Incorporating the old incision is the preferred technique because it decreases the risk of vascular compromise to the soft-tissue sleeve. Care should be taken to elevate full-thickness flaps whenever possible. Medial and lateral full-thickness flaps are used for exposure (**Figure 1**). The incision can be extended proximally and distally to gain access to the entire extensor mechanism.

FIGURE 2

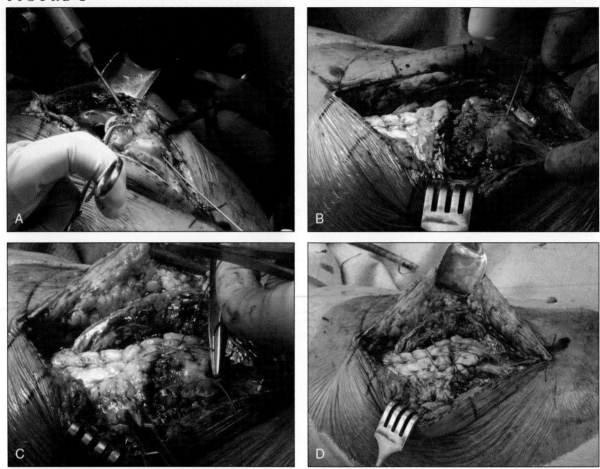

Intraoperative photographs show repair of a patellar tendon rupture with avulsion from the inferior pole of the patella. **A**, A 2- or 3-mm drill bit is used to create two parallel vertical tunnels through the patella. **B**, Heavy nonabsorbable suture is passed through the bone tunnels and sutured to the infrapatellar tendon stump. **C**, Suture is tensioned as tight as possible over the bone bridge with the knee in full extension. **D**, Additional suture is used to augment the repair.

SELECTED SURGICAL TECHNIQUES
Repair of Patellar Tendon Disruption

With type II periprosthetic patellar fractures involving infrapatellar tendon rupture or inferior pole avulsion, primary repair is always attempted to ensure apposition of the torn tendon ends. If the inferior pole of the patella is avulsed, the preferred technique is to excise the avulsed bone fragment and repair the tendon end to the superior patellar fragment. Repair is achieved by the creation of two parallel tunnels through the patellar bone; this can be accomplished with a 2- or 3-mm drill bit (**Figure 2,** *A*). A heavy No. 5 nonabsorbable suture is passed through the tunnels and sutured to the infrapatellar tendon stump (**Figure 2,** *B*). If possible, the suture is woven through native tendon using a Krackow technique. The suture is tensioned in full extension as tight as possible and tied over a bone bridge at the superior patellar pole (**Figure 2,** *C*). The repair is augmented

FIGURE 3

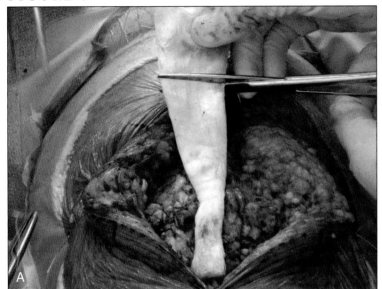

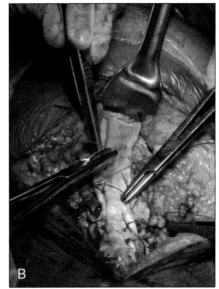

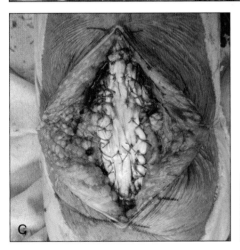

Intraoperative photographs show grafting procedure after completion of the primary tendon repair. **A**, Achilles tendon allograft is sized and trimmed to appropriate length. **B**, The allograft tendon is sutured to the underlying extensor mechanism. **C**, Completed extensor mechanism repair. This should be stable to range of motion.

with the use of No. 1 nonabsorbable suture in an interrupted figure-of-8 technique (**Figure 2**, *D*).

Once the primary repair is completed, the Achilles tendon allograft is prepared. The fresh-frozen allograft tendon is thawed by soaking in antibiotic-impregnated saline solution. The allograft is prepared by excising the calcaneal bone block. The allograft tendon is then sized and trimmed to the length appropriate for the reconstruction (**Figure 3**, *A*). The graft is then sutured to the underlying extensor mechanism (**Figure 3**, *B*). Care

should be taken to perform the repair with the knee in full extension. The allograft tendon is used to "bridge" the primary repair site. The allograft is attached to the underlying extensor mechanism with No. 2 nonabsorbable sutures in an interrupted fashion. Enough tension should be applied to the allograft to keep it taut and unwrinkled. The proximal portion of the repair is extended to the quadriceps tendon, and the distal portion of the repair is extended to the level of the tibial tubercle. Augmentation of the repair into the proximal

FIGURE 4

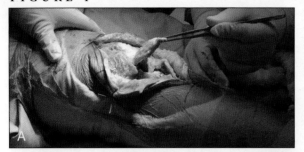

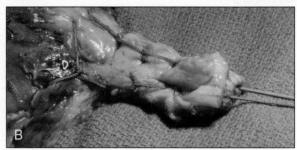

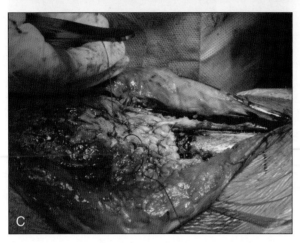

Intraoperative photographs show repair of a patellar tendon rupture from the tibial tubercle. **A**, The ruptured patellar tendon. **B**, Heavy nonabsorbable suture is woven through the native tendon using a Krackow technique. **C**, Repair is achieved by direct attachment to the tibial tubercle through drill holes in the bone.

tibia may be performed with the aid of suture anchors, although this is often not necessary for infrapatellar tendon ruptures proximal to the midtendon region. The completed extensor mechanism repair should be stable to range of motion (**Figure 3**, *C*). Closure is performed with No. 2 braided absorbable suture for the subcutaneous tissue and staples for the skin. The use of a drain is left to the discretion of the surgeon.

Avulsion From the Tibial Tubercle

To repair a patellar tendon that has been avulsed from the tibial tubercle, the incision is extended distally, to the proximal tibia just distal to the tibial tubercle. Care should be taken to elevate full-thickness flaps. Medial and lateral full-thickness flaps are used for exposure. The tendon rupture or avulsion is identified and exposed (**Figure 4**, *A*). Primary repair is attempted to ensure apposition of native tendon to the tibial tubercle. A heavy No. 5 nonabsorbable suture is woven through the

native tendon using a Krackow technique (**Figure 4**, *B*). Repair is achieved by direct attachment to the tibial tubercle (**Figure 4**, *C*); this can be accomplished with a 2- or 3-mm drill bit.

The proximal part of the tibia is prepared for insertion of the calcaneal bone block. A small saw is used to make the osteotomy (**Figure 5**, *A*). Care must be taken to avoid iatrogenic periprosthetic fracture. A rectangular/trapezoidal cavity 2.5 cm long × 1.5 cm wide × 1 cm deep in the proximal part of the tibia is created. The site of the osteotomy is slightly distal and medial to the original insertion site of the patellar tendon. An osteotome is used to lift out the unwanted bone (**Figure 5**, *B*).

The Achilles tendon allograft is then prepared. The calcaneal bone block is cut to match the rectangular/trapezoidal space created in the proximal tibia (**Figure 6**, *A*). A keystone is created to maximize friction fit and bony contact. The bone block is gently impacted into the proximal tibia. Two 3.5-mm screws are used,

FIGURE 5

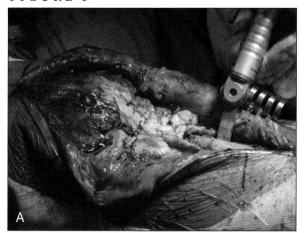 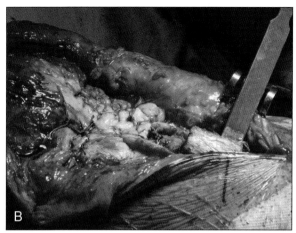

Preparation of the tibia for bone block procedure. **A,** The proximal part of the tibia is prepared for the insertion of calcaneal bone. The osteotomy is performed just distal to the repair site. **B,** An osteotome is used to carefully lift out the unwanted cortical bone. Care must be taken to avoid iatrogenic fracture of the tibial shaft.

which are angled in different planes to avoid the tibial component and lessen the possibility of stress-riser formation (**Figure 6,** *B*). The use of intraoperative fluoroscopy is recommended during the fixation of the allograft bone (**Figure 6,** *C*). The Achilles tendon is then draped over the infrapatellar tendon and patellar bone to the level of the quadriceps tendon. The knee should be positioned in full extension. The allograft is attached to the underlying extensor mechanism with No. 2 nonabsorbable sutures in an interrupted fashion. Enough tension should be applied to the allograft to keep it taut and unwrinkled. The proximal portion of the repair is extended to the quadriceps tendon, and the distal portion of the repair is extended to the level of the tibial tubercle. The completed repair should be stable in flexion (**Figure 6,** *D*). Closure is performed with No. 2 braided absorbable suture for the subcutaneous tissue and staples for the skin. The use of a drain is left to the discretion of the surgeon.

Patellar Fracture

To repair a type IIIb periprosthetic patellar fracture (ie, a periprosthetic patellar fracture with poor remaining bone stock and an intact extensor mechanism), exposure of the extensor mechanism is performed as described previously. Tissue around the patella should be débrided to expose the loose patellar implant and patellar fracture. Débridement of the lateral gutter is often necessary to mobilize the patella. Lateral release can be performed to allow eversion of the patella. The knee should be placed in extension when everting the patella to minimize stress on the fracture and the patellar tendon attachment. The patellar component is removed (**Figure 7,** *A*). Care must be taken to preserve native bone and prevent further displacement of the fracture fragments. Any loose fragments of cement, polyethylene, or necrotic bone are excised. The joint is irrigated copiously with pulsatile lavage, and the patellar fragments of fibrous scar and devitalized bone are débrided.

The patellar bed is then prepared. First, the patella is sized with available templates (**Figure 7,** *B*). Once the size is determined, the patellar remnant is prepared using special patellar hemispherical reamers (**Figure 7,** *C*). The reamers are intended to débride the bone to incite bleeding and shape the bed for the trabecular component for maximum bone-to-implant contact (**Figure 7,** *D*). The implant is then seated into the prepared cancellous bed. The existing patellar shell of bone is used to assess position of the augment. The trabecu-

FIGURE 6

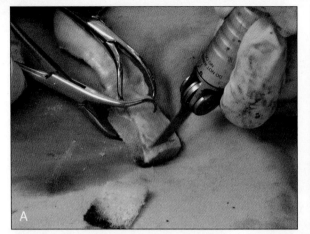

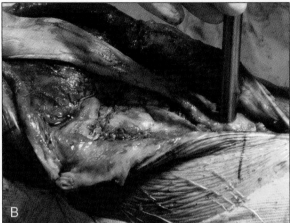

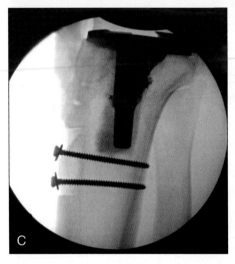

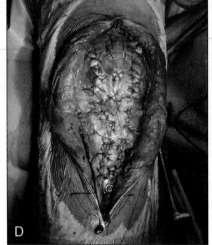

Grafting procedure. **A**, The calcaneal bone block is cut to match the rectangular/trapezoidal cavity that was created in the proximal tibia. **B**, The bone block is fixed to the proximal tibia with 3.5-mm screws. The screws are placed at different angles to avoid the formation of a stress riser. **C**, Intraoperative fluoroscopy is used during fixation of the allograft bone block into the tibia. **D**, The completed tendon graft is tensioned in extension and should be stable in flexion. (Courtesy of Orthopaedia, http://www.orthopaedia.com.)

lar metal implant is fixed to the remaining bone and soft tissue using nonabsorbable sutures through the peripheral holes on the implant (**Figure 7**, *E*). The sutures can be passed through bone with the aid of 1.6- or 2.0-mm drill bits and available suture passers. Incorporation of the fragments into the suture construct is preferred. The trabecular metal implant is used as a scaffolding to fix the fragments together. The final construct should be stable and have intimate contact with the underlying bony fragments. A matching three-peg polyethylene patellar component is then cemented into the trabecular metal augment (**Figure 7**, *F* and *G*). Normal patellar tracking is key in preventing undue stress on the con-

struct. Patellar tracking can be optimized with the use of lateral release.

Repair of the medial retinaculum is performed in the standard technique using No. 1 braided absorbable suture. The subcutaneous tissue and skin are closed using 2-0 braided absorbable suture and staples, respectively. Preoperative and postoperative radiographs reveal reconstitution of the patellar anatomy (**Figure 8**).

POSTOPERATIVE MANAGEMENT

Postoperative management is critical to the success of extensor mechanism reconstruction using allograft tissue and/or a trabecular metal augment patella. The knee

FIGURE 7

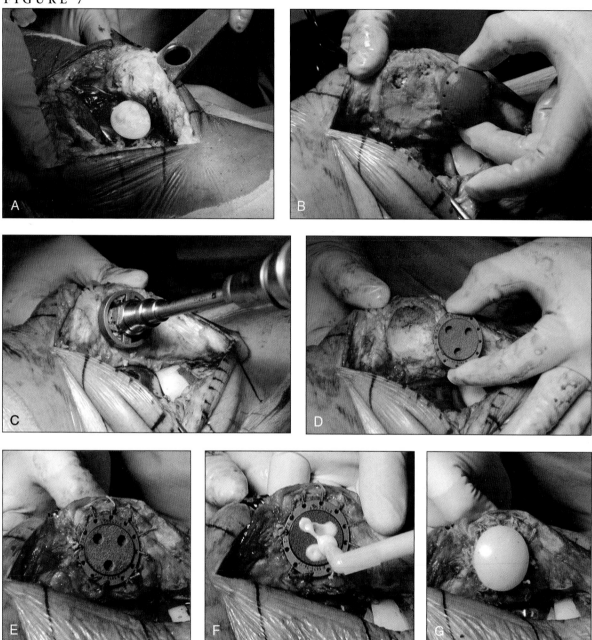

Repair of a fractured patella with a grossly loose patellar component. **A**, Type IIIb patellar fracture. **B**, The patella is sized with available templates. A patellar component is selected that will have good peripheral bone coverage. **C**, Reamers are used to prepare the patella. **D**, A concave surface of bleeding cancellous bone is ideal to receive the trabecular patellar component. **E**, The trabecular metal implant is fixed to the native patella using nonabsorbable suture through drill holes. **F**, Doughy cement is placed on the surface of the trabecular metal augment. **G**, A matching three-peg polyethylene patellar component is cemented onto the augment.

FIGURE 8

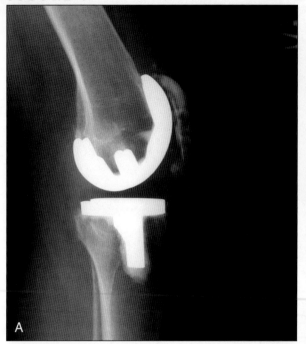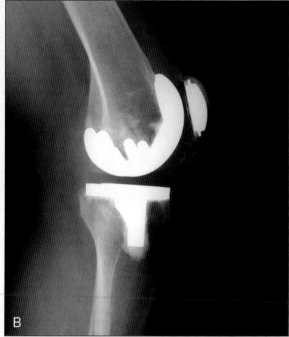

Lateral radiographs of a knee with a periprosthetic patellar fracture. **A**, The fracture before revision surgery. **B**, The knee after revision with a trabecular metal augment patella.

FIGURE 9

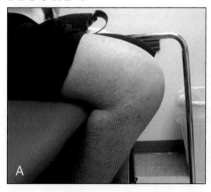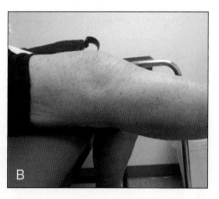

Clinical photographs show full knee flexion (**A**) and active extension (**B**) achieved after reconstruction.

is immobilized in full extension postoperatively with the use of a hinged knee brace. The brace is kept locked in full extension for 3 to 4 weeks. Non–weight-bearing ambulation is recommended for 4 weeks. Gradual range of motion is begun at 3 to 4 weeks postoperatively. The hinged knee brace is unlocked at 4 weeks, with the extension stop initially set at 60°. A gradual increase in flexion is allowed weekly for the following 3 weeks. Typically, passive flexion is increased to 10° each subsequent week until passive flexion is greater than 90°. Most patients will regain preinjury flexion without the need for manipulation under anesthesia (MUA). However, if

MUA becomes necessary, it is advised that it not be attempted for the first 7 to 8 weeks postoperatively to prevent rerupture. Weight bearing is advanced at 4 weeks postoperatively to 50% and then gradually increased to full weight bearing at 8 weeks postoperatively. The brace is discontinued when passive flexion to 90° is achieved. Excellent active range of motion can be achieved with these techniques (**Figure 9**). However, residual extensor weakness can be expected, especially with stair-climbing activities.

REFERENCES

1. Cadambi A, Engh GA: Use of a semitendinosus tendon autogenous graft for rupture of the patellar ligament after total knee arthroplasty: A report of seven cases. *J Bone Joint Surg Am* 1992;74(7):974-979.

2. Lynch AF, Rorabeck CH, Bourne RB: Extensor mechanism complications following total knee arthroplasty. *J Arthroplasty* 1987;2(2):135-140.

3. Rand JA, Morrey BF, Bryan RS: Patellar tendon rupture after total knee arthroplasty. *Clin Orthop Relat Res* 1989;244:233-238.

4. Zehntner MK, Ganz R: Internal fixation of supracondylar fractures after condylar total knee arthroplasty. *Clin Orthop Relat Res* 1993;293:219-224.

5. Ortiguera C, Berry D: Patellar fracture after total knee arthroplasty. *J Bone Joint Surg Am* 2002;84(4):532-540.

6. Dobbs RE, Hanssen AD, Lewallen DG, Pagnano MW: Quadriceps tendon rupture after total knee arthroplasty: Prevalence, complications, and outcomes. *J Bone Joint Surg Am* 2005;87(1):37-45.

7. Emerson RH Jr, Head WC, Malinin TI: Extensor mechanism reconstruction with an allograft after total knee arthroplasty. *Clin Orthop Relat Res* 1994;303:79-85.

8. Crossett LS, Sinha RK, Sechriest VF, Rubash HE: Reconstruction of a ruptured patellar tendon with Achilles tendon allograft following total knee arthroplasty. *J Bone Joint Surg Am* 2002;84(8):1354-1361.

9. Burnett RS, Berger RA, Paprosky WG, Della Valle CJ, Jacobs JJ, Rosenberg AG: Extensor mechanism allograft reconstruction after total knee arthroplasty: A comparison of two techniques. *J Bone Joint Surg Am* 2004;86-A(12):2694-2699.

10. Jaureguito JW, Dubois CM, Smith SR, Gottlieb LJ, Finn HA: Medial gastrocnemius transposition flap for the treatment of disruption of the extensor mechanism after total knee arthroplasty. *J Bone Joint Surg Am* 1997;79(6):866-873.

11. Emerson RH Jr, Head WC, Malinin TI: Reconstruction of patellar tendon rupture after total knee arthroplasty with an extensor mechanism allograft. *Clin Orthop Relat Res* 1990;260:154-161.

12. Nelson CL, Lonner JH, Lahiji A, Kim J, Lotke PA: Use of a trabecular metal patella for marked patella bone loss during revision total knee arthroplasty. *J Arthroplasty* 2003;18(7, Suppl 1):37-41.

CHAPTER 8

REVISION TOTAL KNEE ARTHROPLASTY FOR INFECTION

ATUL F. KAMATH, MD

JESS H. LONNER, MD

INTRODUCTION

The diagnosis and management of periprosthetic joint infection after total knee arthroplasty (TKA) remains a considerable challenge. Although many studies have reported the incidence of infection after TKA to be less than 1% to 2%, recent studies suggest that infection may be increasing in prevalence[1-3] and may rival mechanical problems as the primary cause of implant failure.[4,5] In a sample of 69,663 Medicare patients undergoing TKA, the infection incidence within 2 years and between 2 and 10 years was 1.55% and 0.46%, respectively.[5] Given the growing number of TKAs being performed in the United States, which has increased from approximately 100,000 in 1990 to 250,000 in 2000 to 650,000 in 2010 and could be as many as 3.48 million in 2030, the prevalence of infection may explode, even with conservative risk estimates.[6]

The understanding of the etiology of periprosthetic knee infections and methodical treatment algorithms has continued to evolve, but the ability to eradicate infections has not changed much over the past few decades. Nonetheless, the ultimate goal of eradicating infection and leaving a pain-free, functional knee joint may be optimized with prompt diagnosis and treatment. Two-stage revision, which is the preferred treatment of most chronic and many acute infections, is discussed in this chapter.

INDICATIONS FOR TWO-STAGE REVISION

Late infections that develop as indolent low-grade sepsis are the primary group treated with two-stage revision TKA. Additionally, early postoperative infections and late but acute hematogenous infections should be treated with staged revision when thorough irrigation and débridement fail to resolve the infection. However, in light of recent data that show a high failure rate of irrigation and débridement even for acute infections[7] and a compromise in the ability to eradicate infection with two-stage revision after failed irrigation and débridement, some surgeons are advocating two-stage revision TKA in the setting of acute infections.[8] Two-stage revision is also recommended for acute infections caused by resistant or highly virulent organisms, infection in an immunocompromised or malnourished host, and infection in patients with soft-tissue deficiency,

---

provided soft-tissue coverage is attainable and the extensor mechanism is intact.[9-17]

DIAGNOSIS

The accurate and timely diagnosis of deep infection after TKA is important for initiating and guiding effective treatment, but occasionally such a diagnosis is elusive.[1,18-20] A thorough history, including the nature and onset of symptoms, and a careful physical examination will often provide insight into the mechanism of implant failure. Overt systemic symptoms (eg, fevers or chills) or localized clinical signs (eg, purulent drainage, erythema, or sinus tracts) of infection are often not present. Radiographs rarely distinguish between septic and aseptic failure (**Figure 1**), but select serologic studies are useful for establishing a diagnosis. Erythrocyte sedimentation rate (ESR) and C-reactive protein (CRP) level are more accurate serologic studies than a peripheral white blood cell count, particularly for late infections.[18,21-23] When used together, the ESR (sensitivity of 0.93 and specificity of 0.83) and CRP level (sensitivity of 0.91 and specificity of 0.86) can reliably indicate the presence or absence of infection after TKA.[22]

Knee aspiration for microbiologic culture and cell count is the most effective method for identifying a deep knee infection after TKA.[21,24-26] Serial aspirations,[27] with the patient off antibiotics for 3 or 4 weeks, may significantly enhance the diagnostic yield of cultures. Recent studies suggest that a white blood cell count greater than 2,500 to 3,120 cells/µL and a neutrophil differential greater than 60% to 65% in the aspirate translates to greater than 95% accuracy in diagnosing periprosthetic joint infection.[21,25,26] Although total body technetium Tc-99m scans are not first-line diagnostic tools, they may be useful in assessing other joints for metachronous infection in a patient with multiple painful prosthetic joints when one joint implant is known to be infected.[28,29] White cell–labeled scans are used infrequently.

Intraoperative frozen section histologic analysis can be useful in identifying occult infection, but errors in tissue sampling and the expertise of the histopathologist examining the tissues can impact the accuracy of the test.[30] To improve the yield and accuracy of frozen section and intraoperative culture, multiple representative tissue samples must be obtained from affected regions of the joint. Tissue from the interface between the pros-

FIGURE 1

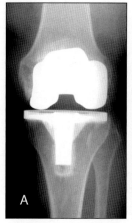
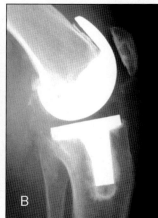

AP (**A**) and lateral (**B**) radiographs of a total knee arthroplasty known to be chronically infected demonstrate no radiographic findings specific for infection.

thesis and bone is usually preferred, but inflamed synovial tissue or granulation tissue also can be useful. Fibrous or fibrin-rich tissue is difficult to interpret and hence should not be used. At least two tissue samples from each knee should be sent, and the five most cellular fields should be analyzed under high-power magnification. The presence of more than ten polymorphonuclear leukocytes (PMNs) per high-power field in five or more fields is almost uniformly consistent with deep periprosthetic infection. The presence of 5 to 9 PMNs per high-power field suggests infection but should be considered in concert with other preoperative diagnostic tests.

Intraoperative cultures are considered the most reliable diagnostic test for infection, but they may be negative in 5% to 8% of acute infections and as many as 20% of chronic or indolent infections.[20] When a strong clinical suspicion for infection exists despite negative preoperative and intraoperative cultures, the knee should be treated as though infected. The accuracy of intraoperative cultures can be improved by withholding preoperative antibiotics from patients with suspected infection in whom the infecting organism is not identified (unlike the protocol when infection is not suspected, in which case preoperative antibiotics are given within 30 to 60 minutes of tourniquet inflation) and sending four or five tissue samples from various affected regions of the knee for aerobic and anaerobic culture to increase the likelihood of identifying not only indolent infection but also polymicrobial infection. After cultures are taken, antibiotics may be administered with deflation of the tourniquet. The choice of antibiotic is based on the results of preoperative aspiration culture. If the infecting organism is not known, a broad-spectrum antibiotic such as vancomycin is administered. Culturing of draining wounds or sinus tracts is not recommended because of the likelihood of false-positive cultures from contaminants.

SURGICAL TECHNIQUE

Two-stage revision is indicated for most late infections.[8,10,16,31] The first stage, implant removal, is followed by an interval during which antibiotic-impregnated cement spacers are in place and intravenous antibiotics are used. The second-stage surgery involves implantation of the revision prosthesis.

First Stage

The index surgical procedure is for implant removal. The procedure should proceed in a systematic and organized manner that enables the surgeon to excise and resect all infected tissues, while preserving viable noninfected bone stock.

Exposure

The surgical approach to a knee with a periprosthetic infection follows the basic tenets of all revision surgery. In the knee with multiple surgical scars, the most lateral incision is used when feasible, provided a standard arthrotomy can be performed through that incision. Sinus tracts within the margins of the skin incision are excised elliptically, down to and including capsular material. Sinus tracts in areas away from the surgical incision are also excised to minimize the risk of further contamination. Extensile exposures are addressed in chapter 3. If the quality or viability of the soft-tissue envelope is questionable—such as with an atrophic skin envelope, a multiply scarred knee, or a knee with large sinus tracts—preoperative consultation with a plastic surgeon is recommended, as rotational muscle flaps may be needed to achieve soft-tissue coverage.

Implant Removal

The femoral component is removed first, using flexible or curved osteotomes, to facilitate exposure of the tibia and prevent femoral debris from falling into the tibial canal. The tibial and patellar components are then removed with a combination of small saw blades and osteotomes. All of the remaining cement is removed, preserving as much viable bone as possible. After all implants have been removed, synovectomy of the posterior aspect of the joint is performed. Although preservation of ligamentous attachments and bone stock is important, thorough débridement of infected or devitalized tissue to clear the infection takes precedence. After removing all cement and necrotic tissue, the knee is irrigated using pulsatile lavage with 6 to 9 L of solution that contains bacitracin and/or polymyxin.

Use of Spacers

Antibiotic-impregnated spacers are used during the period between implant removal/débridement and eventual staged reimplantation. We prefer to use articulating spacers, which allow partial weight bearing, enhance short-term limb function, and enable immediate range of motion, reducing scarring in the gutters and suprapatellar pouch and ultimately facilitating surgical exposure at reimplantation.[9,11,14,32]

The removed femoral component is cleared of adherent bone and soft tissue. Cement on the prosthesis is chipped away using a sharp osteotome (**Figure 2, *A***). The femoral prosthesis is then sterilized in the autoclave. A fresh polyethylene insert of matched size is chosen for the articulating countersurface; the insert thickness must allow relatively balanced flexion and extension spaces. Cement is mixed with high concentrations of antibiotics (eg, 3 g of vancomycin mixed with either 3.6 g of tobramycin or 240 mg of gentamicin per 40 g of polymethyl methacrylate) to provide a high localized dose of broad-spectrum antibiotics. The cement is hand-mixed, as the presence of bubbles in the cement improves antibiotic elution and cement strength is not important at this stage. When it has reached a doughy state, the cement-antibiotic mixture is applied to the undersurfaces of the sterilized femoral component and polyethylene tibial insert (**Figure 2, *B***). An appropriately sized polyethylene tibial component is loosely implanted first, followed by the femoral component,

FIGURE 2

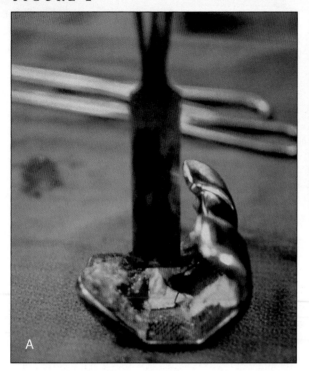

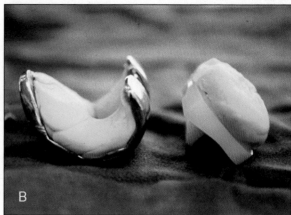

Photographs show preparation of a total knee arthroplasty prosthesis for reimplantation. **A,** An osteotome is used to chip cement off the removed femoral prosthesis before autoclave sterilization. **B,** The underlying surfaces of the sterilized femoral component and a fresh polyethylene tibial insert are coated with a mixture of Palacos cement (Zimmer, Warsaw, IN) and high concentrations of antibiotics.

leaving the cement mantle around each component several millimeters thick (**Figure 3**).

An alternative to dynamic articulating spacers is nonarticulating antibiotic spacer blocks, with similar concentrations of antibiotics per unit of polymethyl methacrylate. The tibia is first capped with a disk of cement, with a small central knob that extends into the débrided metaphyseal defect that had accommodated the previous tibial keel and cement. Appropriate sizing of the tibial disk is important; it must be thick enough to provide a stable base and narrow enough to allow capsular closure, and it must provide enough underlying cancellous and cortical support to minimize subsidence and to protect the trabecular bone from compressing and collapsing during weight bearing. The contour and size of the femoral spacer are equally important. The femoral spacer should be no more than approximately 1 cm thick anteriorly, and the anterior flange should taper proximally to facilitate capsular closure. The femoral spacer is curved distally and posteriorly around the distal femoral condyles (**Figure 4**).

Wound Closure

Wound closure is performed using monofilament suture in a running fashion to minimize knots and braids, which can harbor bacteria. A closed suction drain is not used because it has been shown to reduce the effective dose of local antibiotics.[31] Postoperatively, the patient is allowed protected weight bearing in a brace. When articulating spacers are used, gentle range of motion is encouraged.

Second Stage
Timing of Procedure

Implantation of the revision components is performed when four criteria are met.[33] First, the CRP level should return to normal or near-normal range after a period of antibiotic discontinuation, and the ESR should be within or trending toward normal limits. Second, the underlying cause of infection, if identified, must be adequately addressed; this also includes resolution of infections at remote sites. Third, the health of immunocompromised, malnourished, and medically unstable

FIGURE 3

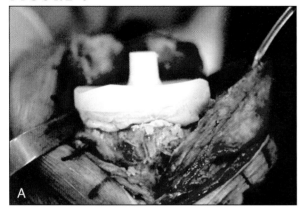

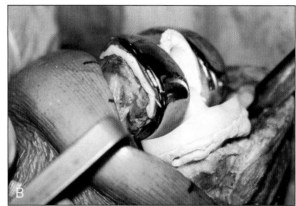

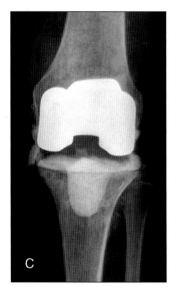

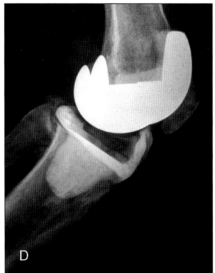

Use of articulating spacers. **A,** Intraoperative photograph shows the tibial spacer inserted into the keel defect and onto the surface of the proximal tibia. The cement is in the doughy stage to avoid pressurization of cement within the trabecular bone. **B,** Intraoperative photograph shows the articulating spacer in place. AP (**C**) and lateral (**D**) radiographs show an articulating spacer in place.

patients should be optimized before reimplantation surgery. Finally, the soft-tissue envelope must be fully healed. Careful assessment of the vascular status of the limb ensures that the risk of wound breakdown is minimized following revision surgery. In general, we prefer to wait 3 months before implanting the revision components, although others have had success performing reimplantation/revision TKA at 6 weeks, provided the criteria are satisfied.

Exposure

At the time of reimplantation, any rotational muscle flaps present are elevated carefully to avoid compromise of the vascular pedicles. After arthrotomy, a thorough synovectomy and excision of scar tissue and pseudocapsule are performed. The tissues are grossly assessed at this point and cultures are sent; histologic analysis using frozen section is less helpful at this stage but can be used, based on clinical suspicion. Lateral retinacular and proximal releases may enhance exposure and allow subluxation of the patella; patellar eversion is not necessary in most revision TKA procedures. The spacer blocks (static or dynamic/articulating) are removed, and further soft-tissue and osseous débridement is performed across intramedullary and extramedullary spaces and surfaces (**Figure 5**). Pulsatile lavage of the knee is per-

FIGURE 4

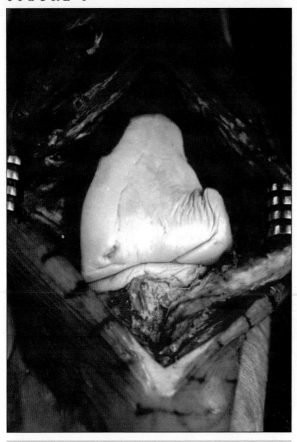

Intraoperative photograph shows a static cement spacer in place.

FIGURE 5

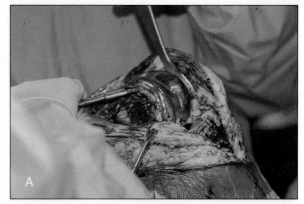

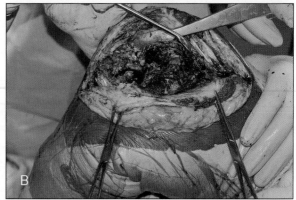

Intraoperative photographs show preparation of a knee for reimplantation. **A,** The articulating spacers can be removed after the cement-bone interface is demarcated. **B,** After removing the spacers, a thorough débridement of soft tissues and bone is once again performed if needed.

formed to define further the extent of bone loss and margins of nonviable soft tissues.

Reimplantation

Reimplantation then proceeds in a stepwise fashion. The tibia is addressed first, to establish a stable platform from which femoral component rotation and gap balance can be determined. Referencing from the endosteal surfaces of the diaphyses is a reproducible and accurate method of preparing the proximal tibia and distal femur. Diaphyseal-engaging intramedullary reamers are used to size the canals for press-fit stems. The appropriately sized reamer can be used as a guide upon which a tibial cutting block is mounted, so that the tibial metaphysis can be resected perpendicular to the tibial mechanical axis.

After the tibial cut surface has been prepared, alignment is confirmed with an extramedullary rod. The trial tray and stem are assembled; a component with offset may be helpful to maximize coverage and avoid overhang of the tibial tray. Once the appropriate trial is set up, including any necessary offset, a keel punch or burr is used to clear bone and to align the tray with the medial third of the tibial tubercle. The trial is left in place during femoral preparation.

Sequential reaming of the femoral canal is performed until the diaphyseal endosteum is engaged. Usually, only a skim cut of the distal femur is necessary to freshen up the bone ends. The orientation of the distal femur can be determined by mounting a cutting guide at the appropriate fixed valgus angle (often between 5° and 7°) on the reamer or trial stem, which is inserted in the femoral canal.

The joint line should be restored to 20 to 25 mm from the medial femoral epicondyle; distal augments in the order of 5 to 10 mm are often necessary to position the femoral component appropriately and reestablish the joint line. Restoration of the joint line and appropriate implantation of components in proper rotational and axial alignment are critical to optimize performance, restore appropriate kinematics, and enhance patellar tracking. Metal augments, not allograft, are used to address bone loss in revisions for septic failure because of a concern that allograft may be more likely to become infected in the presence of persistent infection.

The size of the femoral component is selected to equalize the flexion and extension gaps after the joint line has been restored with appropriate distal augments. The femoral size options may be limited, in part, by the size of the tibial component. Anterior-posterior, chamfer, and box cutting guides are mounted on the intramedullary reamer or trial stem with provisional distal augments applied to ensure that the depth of the box resection and the chamfer cuts are appropriate.

With the knee flexed 90°, the femoral guide is externally rotated, referencing it off the cut tibial surface and manually tensioning the ligaments to reestablish a rectangular flexion space. The transverse axis of the cutting block should be parallel to the transepicondylar axis. Femoral offset options may improve the position of the femoral component and normalize the flexion gap and patellofemoral space. Posterior augments are often required to restore posterior condylar offset and ensure appropriate femoral component rotation.

Constraint

The decision regarding implant constraint is based primarily on the integrity of the collateral ligaments and implant stability with the trial components in place. An unlinked but constrained prosthesis is selected if residual soft-tissue instability exists after attempts to balance the soft tissues with the trials in place. If complete incompetence of one or both collateral ligaments exists, a rotating-hinge prosthesis may be selected. If extensive resection of the distal femur or proximal tibia is necessary for chronic osteomyelitis, a hinged prosthesis with distal femoral or proximal tibial bulk augments is used.

Patellar Resurfacing

The decision to resurface the patella depends on the quality and thickness of the residual bone. Pseudomeniscus and fibrous tissue are débrided from the surface and periphery of the patella. The patella is resurfaced if a 10- to 15-mm thickness of viable bone stock remains; the remnant is left as a bony shell if it is too thin or has evidence of osteonecrosis. Leaving a bony shell is associated with a moderate incidence of anterior knee discomfort; however, resurfacing of an excessively thin or osteonecrotic patella can result in fracture or dissociation of the patellar component. The introduction of trabecular metal has allowed resurfacing of patellae between 4 and 10 mm thick, which otherwise would be considered too thin for resurfacing.

Implantation

After satisfactory trialing, the bony surfaces are prepared for implantation. We typically prefer to cement the condylar surfaces of the tibial and femoral components, including the tibial keel, and use uncemented, press-fit stems (**Figure 6**); however, if the bone is severely osteoporotic with capacious canals, we use cemented stems. At this stage, a low concentration of antibiotics (typically 1.2 g of tobramycin or 500 mg of vancomycin per 40 g of cement) is mixed into the cement to achieve antibiotic delivery without compromising cement strength. The final components are cemented into position (**Figure 7**).

SURGICAL PEARLS

- For stiff knees, proximal releases such as a quadriceps snip are preferred to tibial tubercle osteotomy at the time of implant extraction. A tibial tubercle osteotomy is potentially useful at the time of reimplantation but should be avoided at the time of implant extraction because of the risk of infected nonunion of the tibial tubercle and because the presence of hardware may compromise the ability to completely eradicate the infection.

FIGURE 6

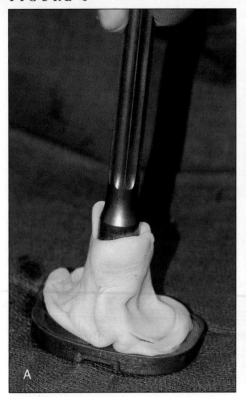

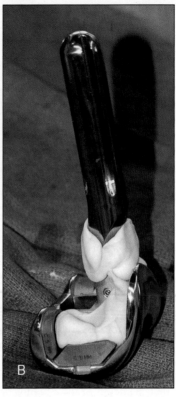

When using press-fit stems, the cement-antibiotic mixture should be applied directly to the metaphyseal segment of the implant to ensure that cement does not extend into the canal. Photographs show correct application to the tibial (**A**) and femoral (**B**) components.

- At the time of spacer implantation, caution must be taken to not pressurize the cement into the trabeculae of the metaphyseal bone. The doughy cement is laid gently onto the bony surfaces, irrigated with water, and backed off periodically to minimize interdigitation of the cement and cancellous bone. As the cement cures, the knee is brought through an arc of motion several times to ensure preservation of appropriate soft-tissue tension. Overdistension of the extension space must be avoided, as this may stretch the collateral ligaments and potentially render them incompetent at the time of revision arthroplasty. Conversely, undertensioning may cause subluxation or dislocation of the polyethylene insert. The latter problems can be avoided by using an all-polyethylene insert with a central keel as the tibial bearing.
- When inserting antibiotic-impregnated cement dowels into the medullary canals during the intervening spacer block stage, it is important to ensure that the dowels are

thinner than the inner canal dimensions to avoid dowel incarceration in the femoral or tibial canals. It is also prudent to check the fit of the dowels during the cement polymerization process. We prefer cement dowels to beads on a metal wire or heavy suture because the beads can become entrapped by abundant fibrous tissue or organized clot that eventually fills the canals.
- The skim cut of the tibial surface at time of reimplantation is usually made at a right angle to the axis of the tibial shaft; however, occasionally an oblique cut is made to accommodate an oblique deformity. A freehand cut may be preferred to freshen up the surface of the proximal tibia, when it is difficult to slide the cutting instrument under the scarred patellar tendon. The alternative is to pin the guide superficial to the patellar tendon and cut around it, but the guide is less stable with this technique, which may lead to a certain amount of error and risk to the patellar tendon.
- The incidence of recurrent infection has not been

proved to be related to whether cemented or uncemented stems are used, but if reinfection develops, press-fit stems are easier to remove. When press-fitting the stems, it is useful to apply cement that has reached a doughy consistency directly to the undersurface of each component, to avoid deposition into the medullary canals. The medullary trabecular surfaces are also coated with cement, leaving a space for passage of the stem.

- Antibiotic-impregnated polymethyl methacrylate premixed with tobramycin (1.2 g tobramycin per 40 g of cement) has been shown to significantly reduce the risk of recurrent infection without compromising the mechanical strength of the cement. If an antibiotic is being added at the time of surgery instead of premixed cement being used, the antibiotic powder should be mixed with the powder of the cement polymer before adding the liquid monomer.

POSTOPERATIVE CARE

Antibiotics are continued empirically until the definitive culture results return, usually in 3 to 5 days. If intraoperative cultures are unexpectedly positive, consultation with an infectious disease specialist is indicated and continuation of antibiotics for at least 6 weeks should be considered, unless deemed a contaminant.

The surgical wound is assessed on postoperative day 1 or 2. If it appears viable and drainage is minimal, then range-of-motion exercises can commence. If wound drainage persists after physical therapy is initiated, the knee is once again wrapped with a compressive dressing and immobilized. In most cases, drainage will stop after 24 to 48 hours of immobilization. If drainage persists despite immobilization, the patient is returned to the operating room for irrigation and débridement of the deep knee wound and joint exploration. Closure is then once again performed in layers. Wound healing takes precedence over motion.

CLINICAL RESULTS

Two-stage revision TKA for late or chronic infection is successful in eradicating infections in 80% to 90% of knees.[8,10-14,16,17,32,34] When the treatment of infection is considered the end point, no clear difference in outcomes is seen in knees with articulating spacers versus knees with static spacers.[9,11,14,32] Articulating spacers are associated with reduced periarticular scarring, which

FIGURE 7

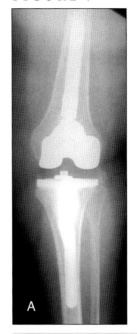
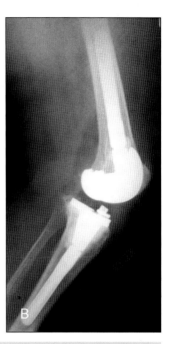

AP (**A**) and lateral (**B**) radiographs after successful revision total knee arthroplasty. The patella was left as a bony shell.

allows easier reimplantation and may result in better ultimate function, although pain scores may be similar.[32] The use of antibiotic-loaded cement at the time of reimplantation may be one of the most effective measures to reduce the risk of recurrent infection. Data are inconclusive regarding the effect of other factors (such as duration of antibiotics, interval to reimplantation, comorbidities, organism virulence, and the use of antibiotic-impregnated spacer blocks) on the reinfection rate.[12]

COMPLICATIONS

Staphylococcus aureus or *S epidermidis* causes most recurrent infections. Although *S epidermidis* is often considered a low-virulence microorganism, it can form a tenacious glycocalyx that resists antibiotics and often adheres to retained tissues despite débridement. The concerning spike in the incidence of antibiotic-resistant organisms, such as methicillin-resistant *S aureus* and *S epidermidis*, has been associated with a recurrent infection rate that may be as high as 24%.[17]

Patients in whom an attempt at staged reimplantation has failed are candidates for salvage procedures, including resection arthroplasty, arthrodesis, and transfemoral amputation. In patients with extensive medical comorbidities who are unable to tolerate multiple surgical procedures, implant resection and débridement without the use of intervening antibiotic spacers may be the best option. These knees may go on to spontaneous autofusion if treated in a cast. Patients with persistent, ongoing infection despite multiple attempted staged revision arthroplasties—as well as those with nonhealing sinus tracts, a compromised soft-tissue envelope, or extensor mechanism incompetence—are not candidates for reimplantation. Staged fusion may be the best alternative in these patients.

Conclusions

Although two-stage revision arthroplasty (including thorough tissue débridement, appropriate and specific parenteral antibiotic therapy, and the use of antibiotic-impregnated cement during an intervening period of 6 to 12 weeks) is the preferred method for treating most late and chronic prosthetic infections, a 10% to 20% recurrent infection rate may be unavoidable. The continued emergence of drug-resistant organisms may, unfortunately, further challenge the success rate.

Eradication of infection and successful restoration of limb function are the goals of revision surgery for the infected TKA. The best chance of success is obtained with expeditious diagnosis and bacterial identification, prompt initiation of surgical and species-specific antibiotic treatment, and maintenance of a viable wound. In the setting of infection, achieving the balance between preservation of bone stock and adequacy of débridement is a challenge that must be addressed individually for each joint. After successful treatment of infection, it is paramount to follow the critical tenets of revision surgery: selecting appropriate incisions, protecting the extensor mechanism, ensuring proper axial and rotational implant alignment, restoring the joint line, and monitoring postoperative rehabilitation.

References

1. Ip D, Yam SK, Chen CK: Implications of the changing pattern of bacterial infections following total joint replacements. *J Orthop Surg (Hong Kong)* 2005;13(2):125-130.

2. Mohanty SS, Kay PR: Infection in total joint replacements: Why we screen MRSA when MRSE is the problem? *J Bone Joint Surg Br* 2004;86(2):266-268.

3. Phillips JE, Crane TP, Noy M, Elliott TS, Grimer RJ: The incidence of deep prosthetic infections in a specialist orthopaedic hospital: A 15-year prospective survey. *J Bone Joint Surg Br* 2006;88(7):943-948.

4. Bozic KJ, Kurtz SM, Lau E, et al: The epidemiology of revision total knee arthroplasty in the United States. *Clin Orthop Relat Res* 2010;468(1):45-51.

5. Kurtz SM, Ong KL, Lau E, Bozic KJ, Berry D, Parvizi J: Prosthetic joint infection risk after TKA in the Medicare population. *Clin Orthop Relat Res* 2010;468(1):52-56.

6. Kurtz S, Ong K, Lau E, Mowat F, Halpern M: Projections of primary and revision hip and knee arthroplasty in the United States from 2005 to 2030. *J Bone Joint Surg Am* 2007;89(4):780-785.

7. Deirmengian C, Greenbaum J, Lotke PA, Booth RE Jr, Lonner JH: Limited success with open debridement and retention of components in the treatment of acute Staphylococcus aureus infections after total knee arthroplasty. *J Arthroplasty* 2003;18(7, Suppl 1):22-26.

8. Sherrell JC, Fehring TK, Odum S, et al: The Chitranjan Ranawat Award: Fate of two-stage reimplantation after failed irrigation and débridement for periprosthetic knee infection. *Clin Orthop Relat Res* 2011;469(1):18-25.

9. Fehring TK, Odum S, Calton TF, Mason JB: Articulating versus static spacers in revision total knee arthroplasty for sepsis: The Ranawat Award. *Clin Orthop Relat Res* 2000;(380):9-16.

10. Goldman RT, Scuderi GR, Insall JN: 2-stage reimplantation for infected total knee replacement. *Clin Orthop Relat Res* 1996;331:118-124.

11. Haddad FS, Masri BA, Campbell D, McGraw RW, Beauchamp CP, Duncan CP: The PROSTALAC functional spacer in two-stage revision for infected knee replacements: Prosthesis of antibiotic-loaded acrylic cement. *J Bone Joint Surg Br* 2000;82(6):807-812.

12. Hanssen AD, Rand JA, Osmon DR: Treatment of the infected total knee arthroplasty with insertion of another prosthesis: The effect of antibiotic-impregnated bone cement. *Clin Orthop Relat Res* 1994;309:44-55.

13. Hirakawa K, Stulberg BN, Wilde AH, Bauer TW, Secic M: Results of 2-stage reimplantation for infected total knee arthroplasty. *J Arthroplasty* 1998;13(1):22-28.

14. Hofmann AA, Kane KR, Tkach TK, Plaster RL, Camargo MP: Treatment of infected total knee arthroplasty using an articulating spacer. *Clin Orthop Relat Res* 1995;321:45-54.

15. Kilgus DJ, Howe DJ, Strang A: Results of periprosthetic hip and knee infections caused by resistant bacteria. *Clin Orthop Relat Res* 2002;404:116-124.

16. Lonner JH, Beck TD Jr, Rees H, Roullet M, Lotke PA: Results of two-stage revision of the infected total knee arthroplasty. *Am J Knee Surg* 2001;14(1):65-67.

17. Mittal Y, Fehring TK, Hanssen A, Marculescu C, Odum SM, Osmon D: Two-stage reimplantation for periprosthetic knee infection involving resistant organisms. *J Bone Joint Surg Am* 2007;89(6):1227-1231.

18. Austin MS, Ghanem E, Joshi A, Lindsay A, Parvizi J: A simple, cost-effective screening protocol to rule out periprosthetic infection. *J Arthroplasty* 2008;23(1):65-68.

19. Barrack RL, Aggarwal A, Burnett RS, et al: The fate of the unexpected positive intraoperative cultures after revision total knee arthroplasty. *J Arthroplasty* 2007;22(6, Suppl 2):94-99.

20. Parvizi J, Ghanem E, Menashe S, Barrack RL, Bauer TW: Periprosthetic infection: What are the diagnostic challenges? *J Bone Joint Surg Am* 2006;88(Suppl 4):138-147.

21. Della Valle CJ, Sporer SM, Jacobs JJ, Berger RA, Rosenberg AG, Paprosky WG: Preoperative testing for sepsis before revision total knee arthroplasty. *J Arthroplasty* 2007;22(6, Suppl 2):90-93.

22. Greidanus NV, Masri BA, Garbuz DS, et al: Use of erythrocyte sedimentation rate and C-reactive protein level to diagnose infection before revision total knee arthroplasty: A prospective evaluation. *J Bone Joint Surg Am* 2007;89(7):1409-1416.

23. Niskanen RO, Korkala O, Pammo H: Serum C-reactive protein levels after total hip and knee arthroplasty. *J Bone Joint Surg Br* 1996;78(3):431-433.

24. Duff GP, Lachiewicz PF, Kelley SS: Aspiration of the knee joint before revision arthroplasty. *Clin Orthop Relat Res* 1996;331:132-139.

25. Mason JB, Fehring TK, Odum SM, Griffin WL, Nussman DS: The value of white blood cell counts before revision total knee arthroplasty. *J Arthroplasty* 2003;18(8):1038-1043.

26. Trampuz A, Hanssen AD, Osmon DR, Mandrekar J, Steckelberg JM, Patel R: Synovial fluid leukocyte count and differential for the diagnosis of prosthetic knee infection. *Am J Med* 2004;117(8):556-562.

27. Barrack RL, Jennings RW, Wolfe MW, Bertot AJ: The Coventry Award: The value of preoperative aspiration before total knee revision. *Clin Orthop Relat Res* 1997;345:8-16.

28. Levitsky KA, Hozack WJ, Balderston RA, et al: Evaluation of the painful prosthetic joint: Relative value of bone scan, sedimentation rate, and joint aspiration. *J Arthroplasty* 1991;6(3):237-244.

29. Scher DM, Pak K, Lonner JH, Finkel JE, Zuckerman JD, Di Cesare PE: The predictive value of indium-111 leukocyte scans in the diagnosis of infected total hip, knee, or resection arthroplasties. *J Arthroplasty* 2000;15(3):295-300.

30. Lonner JH, Desai P, Dicesare PE, Steiner G, Zuckerman JD: The reliability of analysis of intraoperative frozen sections for identifying active infection during revision hip or knee arthroplasty. *J Bone Joint Surg Am* 1996;78(10):1553-1558.

31. Lonner JH, Parvizi J: Staged revision of the infected total knee arthroplasty, in Lotke PA, Lonner JH, eds: *Master Techniques in Orthopaedic Surgery: Knee Arthroplasty,* ed 3. Philadelphia, PA, Lippincott Williams & Wilkins, 2009, pp 275-300.

32. Freeman MG, Fehring TK, Odum SM, Fehring K, Griffin WL, Mason JB: Functional advantage of articulating versus static spacers in 2-stage revision for total knee arthroplasty infection. *J Arthroplasty* 2007;22(8):1116-1121.

33. Lonner JH: Identifying ongoing infection after resection arthroplasty and before second-stage reimplantation. *Am J Knee Surg* 2001;14(1):68-71.

34. Haleem AA, Berry DJ, Hanssen AD: Mid-term to long-term followup of two-stage reimplantation for infected total knee arthroplasty. *Clin Orthop Relat Res* 2004;428:35-39.

CHAPTER 9

REVISION TOTAL KNEE ARTHROPLASTY FOR PERIPROSTHETIC FRACTURE

DAVID BACKSTEIN, MD, MED, FRCSC

INTRODUCTION

The number of primary total knee arthroplasty (TKA) procedures performed annually has been rising sharply, with more than 300,000 such procedures currently performed in the United States each year.[1,2] Between 1990 and 2002, the rate of primary TKA implantation in the United States almost tripled, and a similar trend has been observed for revision procedures.[2] The incidence of periprosthetic fracture ranges from 0.3% to 2.5%,[3,4] and given the rise in primary and revision surgery as well as the aging of those TKAs that were implanted over the past 3 to 4 decades, the frequency with which orthopaedic surgeons will face periprosthetic fracture of the knee is likely to rise significantly.

Periprosthetic fractures can occur intraoperatively or postoperatively. Intraoperative fractures may be a result of inadvertent cortical perforations, forceful impaction of components or trials, eccentric placement of femoral box cuts in posterior stabilized implants, or forceful flexion of stiff knees. In a review of more than 17,000 primary TKAs, Alden et al[5] found that intraoperative fracture occurred in 0.39% of cases and was most common in females and on the femoral side. Fractures that are identified intraoperatively during primary or revision arthroplasty should be stabilized and protected by a stem so that range-of-motion exercises can proceed as usual, although weight bearing will likely need to be delayed.[6]

These are usually metaphyseal fractures, which can be adequately fixed with screws and protected by a stem. Autologous bone graft from reamings or other local sites should be added to the fracture site to promote union.

Periprosthetic fractures that occur early in the postoperative phase may result from trauma or intraoperative technical errors, such as the production of stress risers, excessive patellar bone resection, and cortical perforations.[7,8] More commonly, periprosthetic fractures occur in the late postoperative phase as a result of minor trauma with or without associated pathologic bone secondary to osteolysis, osteopenia,[9] rheumatoid arthritis, corticosteroid use, increased age, or female sex.

This chapter reviews the diagnostic, decision-making, and therapeutic features pertinent to revision arthroplasty for periprosthetic fractures around TKAs. The primary focus is on fractures occurring in the postoperative period, which are not amenable to fixation or osteosynthesis using intramedullary nails or plates.

RISK FACTORS
Early Postoperative Periprosthetic Fractures

Intraoperative or early postoperative periprosthetic fractures may be minimized by taking critical preventive measures. In knees with previously placed hardware such as plates and screws, removal of hardware should

Dr. Backstein or an immediate family member is a member of a speakers' bureau or has made paid presentations on behalf of Sanofi-Aventis, Stryker, and Zimmer and serves as a paid consultant to or is an employee of Sanofi-Aventis, Stryker, and Zimmer.

be considered at least 3 months before primary TKA. Alternatively, if the hardware is removed at the same time as the TKA is performed, stems should be used to bypass stress risers.[6] Production of such stress risers may lead to fracture with weight bearing or minimal trauma in the early postoperative phase.

Excessively eccentric placement of the femoral box cut for posterior stabilized femoral components should be avoided. This malposition may cause one condyle to be small and thin, leading to condylar fracture.[10] These fractures are most likely to occur intraoperatively, during placement of trials or the definitive implant, and they mandate fixation. When they occur, these fractures should be stabilized with cancellous screws and protected by a stemmed implant.

In TKA after previous lateral closing wedge high tibial osteotomy, extra-articular deformity and lateral bone loss can cause overly lateral placement of the tibial component or stem. This may result in perforation of the lateral cortex unless care is taken to ensure that the keel is appropriately placed either by using intramedullary tibial cutting guides or taking confirmatory intraoperative radiographs. Similarly, TKA in a knee that has previously undergone a medial closing wedge distal femoral varus osteotomy is prone to medial cortical perforation unless the starting point for intramedullary guides is moved more laterally. In both situations, failure to bypass cortical perforations with stems may result in early postoperative fractures due to cortical stress risers.

The integrity of the anterior femoral cortex may be compromised as a result of perforation by intramedullary instrumentation or from anterior cortical notching. If a significant perforation (>1 cm in diameter) or notching greater than 3 mm does occur, bypassing the stress riser with a stem should be considered,[6] to lessen the likelihood of postoperative fracture.

Revision TKA is fraught with characteristics that potentially lead to mechanical weakening and put the patient at risk for early postoperative fracture. Stemmed components should be used in all revision situations. Guidewires and intraoperative radiographs should be used when any doubt exists regarding reamer placement, to avoid enlarging unrecognized perforations. When a perforation has indeed been recognized, the stem should bypass the defect by two cortical diameters.[11] Intraoperative radiographs obtained with trial stems in place are very helpful for confirmation that cortical perforations or stress risers have been adequately protected with bypassing stems, plates, or bone graft before leaving the operating room.

Late Postoperative Periprosthetic Fractures

Fractures around TKAs that occur late in the postoperative phase are a result of either significant trauma or pathologic bone, with or without loosened implants. The etiology of weakened, pathologic bone is usually osteoporosis or polyethylene debris and subsequent osteolysis. Osteoporosis is most often seen in the elderly, in patients with rheumatoid arthritis, and in patients with chronic steroid use. Osteolysis secondary to polyethylene wear results in areas of weakened bone. Lesions may form small, large, or massive defects; these may be contained or associated with cortical erosion. Less frequently, periprosthetic fractures are seen in association with neurologic disorders such as epilepsy, Parkinson disease, cerebellar ataxia, and myasthenia gravis.[12,13]

CLASSIFICATION

Although numerous classification schemes have been published that describe fracture characteristics and prescribe treatment options for periprosthetic fractures, an ideal, all-encompassing classification system has yet to be published. Most authors would agree that the three critical features that determine ideal treatment of periprosthetic fractures are (1) the location, configuration, and displacement of the fracture; (2) the quality of surrounding bone; and (3) the fixation and alignment of the associated TKA implants. These features are the basis of all modern classification systems of periprosthetic fractures.

The classification shown in **Table 1** has been developed and used at our institution.[6] A femoral periprosthetic fracture is defined as a supracondylar fracture within 15 cm of the femoral prosthesis. A tibial periprosthetic fracture is defined as a tibial fracture within 15 cm of the tibial prosthesis. Fractures are further qualified according to prosthesis stability and bone stock quality as follows: S = stable prosthesis; L = loose prosthesis; g = good bone stock; p = poor bone stock. For example, a femoral periprosthetic fracture located just above a well-fixed component with poor bone stock would be classified as F2 Sp.

TABLE 1 Classification of Periprosthetic Fractures

Type	Characteristics
Femoral	
F1	The fracture is sufficiently distant from the femoral component to provide adequate bone for retrograde nail and locking screws or plate fixation.
F2	The extent of the distal fracture fragment does not provide adequate bone for a retrograde nail or plate fixation and thus revision is indicated. These fractures are usually distal to the most proximal extent of the anterior femoral component flange.
Tibial	
T1	The extent of the proximal fracture fragment is large enough to allow internal fixation with a plate.
T2	The extent of the proximal fracture fragment is not large enough to allow internal fixation, and thus TKA revision is indicated.

INDICATIONS

Revision TKA, as opposed to osteosynthesis, is indicated for the treatment of periprosthetic fractures when the fracture is very close to the prosthesis, usually distal to the most proximal extent of the femoral component flange or proximal to the keel of the tibial component. In this setting, solid fixation is very difficult to achieve using modern plates or an intramedullary nail (**Figure 1**). Even if adequate reduction and fixation is possible, this mode of treatment requires a prolonged period of protected weight bearing that is suboptimal in the elderly patients who commonly sustain these fractures. The ultimate effectiveness of treatment of these fractures is highly dependent on achieving alignment and stability as good as was present before fracture. Furthermore, fixation of very distal fractures is associated with high nonunion or malunion rates[4] (**Figure 2**). This is particularly true when the fracture is associated with comminution and osteoporosis. Accordingly, our practice is to revise rather than attempt to fix periprosthetic

FIGURE 1

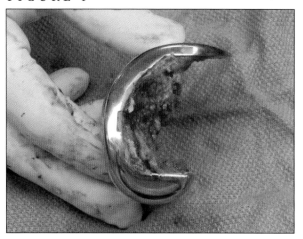

Intraoperative photograph of a femoral component after distal femoral periprosthetic fracture. Note the minimal bone available for fixation.

fractures of the knee that are very close to the femoral or tibial implants, particularly when associated with osteoporosis or comminution in elderly patients, who need to be mobilized early. Fractures best managed with revision arthroplasty include very distal periprosthetic fractures of the femur or very proximal fractures of the femur; fractures around loose components; and fractures associated with severe osteoporosis or osteolytic defects.

Very distal periprosthetic fractures of the femur or very proximal fractures of the tibia are poor candidates for fixation rather than repair because fractures that are immediately adjacent to the femoral or tibial implant do not provide adequate bone for plate or intramedullary nail fixation. These fractures are distal to the proximal extent of the femoral component or proximal to the distal extent of the tibial component. Attempts at fixing such fractures, even if technically possible, are likely to result in a construct that is so tenuous as to prohibit any weight bearing for a prolonged period of time. Clearly, long periods of immobilization are not in the best interests of elderly patients.

When a fracture occurs around a loose TKA implant, both the fracture and the failed implant fixation should be addressed with a single operation. Although it is possible to fix the fracture and reoperate at a later date to deal with the loose implant, this is clearly a suboptimal

FIGURE 2

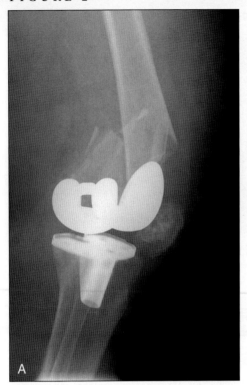
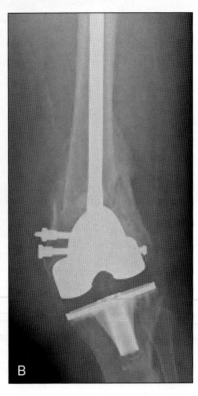

Radiographs of a distal femoral periprosthetic fracture. **A**, Oblique view obtained before treatment with retrograde intramedullary nailing. **B**, AP view after treatment demonstrates valgus malunion.

strategy. In addition to the requirement of a second operation, the fracture fixation hardware will add to the revision TKA complexity. It is therefore preferable to treat fractures around loose implants with a single revision arthroplasty procedure.

When a periprosthetic fracture is associated with severe osteoporosis or osteolytic defects, stable fracture osteosynthesis is likely to be impossible to achieve. Even with modern fixation techniques and implants, large osteolytic defects or severe osteoporosis will compromise fixation and continue to put the TKA at risk for subsequent periprosthetic fracture. For these reasons, we recommend revision TKA in these situations. Using stems, bone grafts, and metallic augments produces a construct that is less likely to suffer subsequent fracture and allows immediate mobilization of the patient.

PREOPERATIVE EVALUATION
Revision TKA surgery for periprosthetic fracture is a complex procedure, and thus a thorough preoperative evalu-

ation is required. Medical optimization with a preoperative evaluation by an internal medicine and/or anesthesia specialist may be indicated, depending on the patient's comorbidities. Although revision TKA surgery is performed under tourniquet control, postoperative transfusion may be required. In preparation, two to four units of packed red blood cells should be made available.

A thorough history of the period leading up to the fracture should be obtained. The presence of prefracture pain, swelling, or instability indicates that there may have been preexisting component loosening. A history of a prefracture effusion and/or pain may also suggest underlying polyethylene wear and osteolysis.

A complete understanding of the fracture pattern, bone quality, and implant fixation is needed before undertaking revision surgery. A complete set of radiographs, including AP, lateral, and oblique views, should be obtained. Further information is acquired by means of CT scanning with metal subtraction software. Although CT is not always a necessity, it can provide a

FIGURE 3

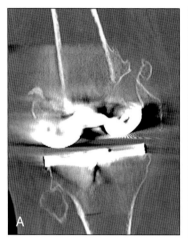 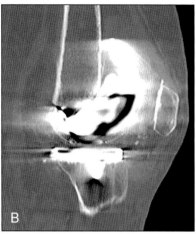

Preoperative coronal (**A**) and sagittal (**B**) CT cuts show a femoral periprosthetic fracture. Note the minimal bone stock available for fracture fixation.

great deal of information about the precise configuration of the fracture as well as the size and quality of remaining bone attachments to the implants (**Figure 3**). Additionally, some basic templating should be done to determine the sizes of components that will be needed.

It is critical to understand the condition of the collateral ligaments, particularly the medial collateral ligament (MCL). If the medial condyle or epicondyle is fractured and displaced, there will be gross instability of the knee unless the fracture can be fixed or the knee is revised to a hinged prosthesis, which compensates for the MCL. Fracture fixation of the medial condyle cannot be easily or reliably accomplished in the presence of osteoporosis, fracture comminution, or revision implants, which preclude placement of large screws or circumferential wires. We therefore recommend having a hinged prosthesis available for these situations. In addition, it is advisable to have structural and morcellized allograft bone available before commencing revision TKA for periprosthetic fracture.

SURGICAL TECHNIQUE

The patient is placed supine on the operating room table. The chosen anesthesia modality should provide ample time to conduct a complex procedure. Either general or regional anesthetics may be used; however, if a regional is chosen for a procedure expected to last more than 2.5 hours, a combined spinal-epidural method is preferable. Preoperative prophylactic antibiotics are administered within 30 minutes of incision. We do not allow the tourniquet time to exceed 120 minutes.

Exposure and Component Removal

The primary TKA skin incision is used for exposure. The skin and subcutaneous tissue are divided, and careful attention is paid to avoid elevation of large subcutaneous flaps. Minimal separation of subcutaneous fascia will maximize blood supply to the skin and help avoid wound complications. A medial parapatellar arthrotomy is conducted. The tibial insertion of the patellar tendon should be protected throughout the operation. Forceful flexion of the knee or eversion of the patella must be avoided. Our practice is to conduct all knee arthroplasty procedures, including revision for periprosthetic fracture, without eversion of the patella. Retropatellar scar and fat are excised to improve visualization of the lateral side of the knee as needed. If there is any suspicion of infection based on history or physical examination, deep tissue is sent for frozen section analysis as well as culture and sensitivity. If these tests do not rule out infection, an antibiotic-loaded cement spacer should be implanted until the infection is ruled out or treated.

The medial and lateral gutters of the knee are cleared of any scar tissue to further facilitate exposure. In our experience, supplemental exposure maneuvers are rarely required in these cases. However, before undertaking this type of surgery, the surgeon should be well acquainted with techniques such as the quadriceps snip, tibial tubercle osteotomy, and V-Y quadricepsplasty (see chapter 3).

Once exposure is achieved, care is taken to minimize disruption of bone fragments until the precise configuration of the fracture is assessed. It is particularly important to gain an early assessment of the status of the medial condyle or epicondyle. If the MCL is incompetent because of fracture of the medial condyle or epicondyle, a hinged prosthesis is likely to be needed unless the medial fracture can be solidly fixed.

Next, the femoral and tibial components are removed. Care should be taken to minimize damage to residual bone. The femoral component is removed first, followed by the tibial side. Removal of the polyethylene liner will help facilitate exposure if there is any difficulty in this regard. The reciprocating saw is an excellent tool to disrupt the implant-cement interface. This can be used on both the femoral and tibial sides. Final loosening of components is accomplished with a cement osteotome.

General Principles

We revise both the femoral and tibial components in almost all cases because it is necessary to achieve proper alignment and balance. Conversion to stemmed implants on both sides is strongly recommended to provide the additional fixation required for a more highly constrained construct.

The tibial side is addressed first. The tibial canal is opened and a guidewire is passed to ensure there are no perforations. Next, hand reaming of the tibial canal is performed until chatter is heard and felt. Using the intramedullary tibial cutting block, the tibial cut is freshened, removing as little bone as possible. At this point, bone defects are noted and a strategy is formulated for bone reconstitution or replacement. Segmental medial or lateral uncontained defects of 20 mm or less that lack a cortical rim are managed with metal augments. Defects larger than 20 mm may require structural allograft. Circumferential defects (involving both the medial and lateral side) may be reconstructed in a similar fashion; however, increased thickness of the polyethylene liner also may be used to reconstitute the joint line. Contained defects that have a maintained cortical rim may be dealt with using morcellized allograft, metal sleeves, or porous metal cones. A tibial baseplate is sized and the rotation is set by aligning the center of the trial component with the middle third of the tibial tubercle. A trial tibial baseplate with the appropriately sized stem is then assembled and inserted.

The femoral side is addressed next. The femoral canal is opened and reamed with hand reamers. With the knee in 90° of flexion, a component is chosen that provides a stable flexion gap and avoids medial-lateral overhang. We use diaphyseal-fitting stems whenever possible because they can both achieve an excellent fit and automatically correct limb alignment. In revision surgery, many landmarks such as the Whiteside line (AP axis) and posterior condylar line are absent, and thus femoral rotation is based on the transepicondylar axis if possible.

Femoral bone defects are dealt with similarly to those on the tibial side. Segmental uncontained defects may be reconstructed with augments up to approximately 20 mm, depending on the revision system used. Circumferential defects may require distal femoral replacement or distal femoral allograft-implant composites (AICs). This will be discussed in detail in the next section.

Femoral Supracondylar Periprosthetic Fractures

In revision TKA for a very distal supracondylar femoral periprosthetic fracture, the tibial side is addressed first. Next, the femoral component is removed by carefully using a reciprocating saw to disrupt the cement-implant junction. The anterior flange is worked on first, followed by the medial and lateral condyles. The reciprocating saw must be kept parallel to the implant and not allowed to diverge into the femoral bone. The posterior condyles and femoral notch are freed from the implant using a straight, flat osteotome of appropriate width. The implant should never be forced off with heavy blows from an impactor or punch. The implant should be freed sufficiently until it can be removed with minimal force and risk to remaining bone.

Once the component has been removed, the fracture pattern and bone quality are assessed. Assessment of the status of the medial condyle is most critical because a fracture that affects the MCL and is not readily repairable with screws or a plate will necessitate the use of a hinged prosthesis. Failure to reconstitute the medial column and the function of the MCL will risk severe instability and dislocation.

The femoral canal is reamed by hand for a diaphyseal-fitting stem. A femoral component size is chosen that

FIGURE 4

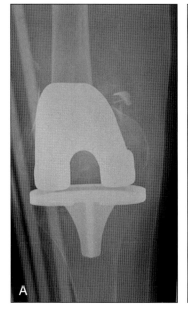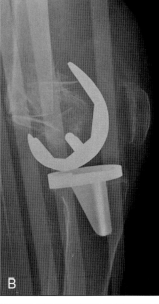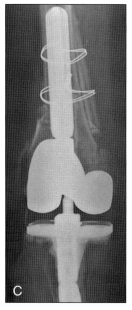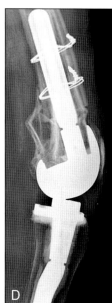

Radiographs of a femoral periprosthetic fracture. Preoperative AP (**A**) and lateral (**B**) views demonstrate significant bone loss. Postoperative AP (**C**) and lateral (**D**) radiographs demonstrate a united distal femoral allograft-implant composite.

will provide an appropriate flexion gap with the knee in 90° of flexion. A trial femoral component and stem are inserted with a trial polyethylene liner of a thickness chosen to provide a stable flexion gap. The knee is then carefully brought into extension and the proximal-distal position of the femoral component is chosen to allow full extension and a stable extension gap.

Once the proximal-distal position of the femoral component has been chosen, the gaps between the patient's native bone and the trial implant represent the bone deficiencies, which must be compensated for. On the femoral side, segmental, uncontained defects of up to 20 mm can usually be dealt with using metallic augments. Larger uncontained defects require a structural allograft. Circumferential defects up to 20 mm can similarly be compensated for using augments on both the medial and lateral side. Circumferential defects larger than 20 mm require an AIC or a distal femoral replacement prosthesis (**Figure 4**).

The decision to choose an AIC over a distal femoral replacement is based on patient age and activity level. Physiologically younger, more active patients who can tolerate a period of non–weight bearing will benefit from the bone reconstitution that an AIC provides. Furthermore, should another revision ever be required, the AIC technique will allow for improved bone stock and a less complex revision procedure. In contrast, elderly, more sedentary patients or those with comorbidities that make a period of non–weight bearing difficult will benefit from the immediate mobility that a distal femoral replacement provides (**Figure 5**). Also, because these patients arc less likely to require further surgery in the future, restoring bone stock is less of a priority.

Tibial Periprosthetic Fractures

Tibial periprosthetic fractures are less common than femoral fractures, but they can be equally challenging to treat when they are very proximally located. Fractures just below the level of the baseplate or involving a single side of the tibial plateau are very difficult to fix reliably using plates because of the presence of a keel and poor bone quality.

FIGURE 5

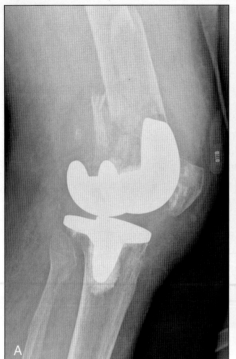
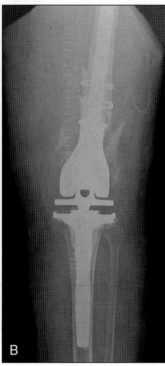

Radiographs of a femoral periprosthetic fracture with significant bone loss in an elderly patient. **A**, Preoperative lateral view. **B**, Postoperative AP view after treatment with distal femoral–replacement type of revision total knee prosthesis.

When treating these fractures with revision TKA, the surgical principles are similar to those already outlined. The tibial baseplate is carefully removed using a reciprocating saw and osteotomes. Particular attention must be paid to protection of the extensor mechanism at the level of the patellar tendon and tibial tubercle. To avoid the possibility of avulsion, the patellar tendon must not be forcefully everted or retracted. Furthermore, the tibial tubercle must not be fractured from the remaining proximal tibia.

Once the baseplate has been removed, the tibial canal is reamed for a diaphyseal-fitting stem. The level of the joint line is chosen based on anatomic markers and radiographic measurements. A stemmed trial tibial baseplate is inserted, and the bone defects are assessed. Segmental defects up to approximately 20 mm can be compensated for using metallic augments, but structural allograft is needed for larger defects. Circumferential defects up to 40 to 45 mm may be dealt with using augments on both the medial and lateral side in addi-

tion to thicker polyethylene liners. For circumferential defects larger than 45 mm, a tibial AIC or proximal tibial replacement will be needed, as a revision baseplate will otherwise teeter on the tibial diaphysis, which is clearly not a stable construct.

Allograft-Implant Composite Technique

The allograft bone chosen for use in an AIC should be from the same side of the body and approximately the same size as the patient's own femur or tibia. Avoiding an oversized allograft is important, as excessive bulk may cause difficulty with wound closure.

On the femoral side, the epicondyles and attached collateral ligaments are removed from the remaining host bone so that they may be attached to the allograft once it has been implanted. The residual diaphyseal-metaphyseal bone is cut to create one side of a step-cut junction. This step cut should be fashioned so that it incorporates adequate external rotation for the proper patellar tracking once the AIC has been implanted. The longer end of the step cut should be on the side of the more viable host bone, to minimize loss of viable bone.[6,14]

The AIC is fashioned on a separate allograft preparation side table (**Figure 6**). The femoral allograft epicondyles are removed with an oscillating saw. The distal end of the graft is cut and shaped using revision TKA cutting jigs. The allograft canal is reamed to accept the same-sized stem, which achieved a press fit in the host diaphyseal bone. The knee is balanced in flexion by the combination of tibial baseplate position and the femoral component, combined with an appropriate-thickness polyethylene insert. For the tibia, the joint line location is reconstituted by rebuilding the proximal tibia to an appropriate height based on standard radiographic measurements such as the distance from the tip of the fibula or medial epicondyle.

An initial step cut is made in the diaphysis of the allograft, complementary to the step cut in the patient's host bone. The graft length is determined by balancing the flexion and extension gaps and gradually shortening the length of the graft until the knee is stable in both flexion and extension.

After being appropriately sized and shaped, the allograft bone is thoroughly cleansed and dried on the side table. For femoral grafts, heavy nonabsorbable sutures are passed through drill holes in the area of the epicondyles for attachment of host epicondyles. Cement with prophylactic-dose antibiotic is mixed, and the implant is cemented into the allograft on the allograft preparation table. Next, the AIC is press-fit into the host using the implant stem. Placement of any cement at the host-graft junction is avoided to allow for host-allograft union. Fixation of the graft to the host is provided by the press-fit of stems, and rotatory stability is gained from the step cut. If further fixation is needed, it may be added using a cortical strut allograft at the junction site. Cement is not used in the host intramedullary canal at all. This allows for easy removal in the situation of subsequent revision, if necessary.

For femoral grafts, the knee is placed in 90° of flexion, and the host epicondyles are fixed tightly and as anteriorly as possible to the allograft bone with the nonabsorbable sutures that were previously placed. The degree of implant constraint required is determined by assessing varus and valgus stresses at the tibiofemoral articulation. A standard posterior-stabilized articulation

FIGURE 6

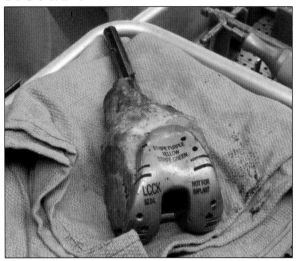

Photograph of allograft-implant composite with trial components in place. Note that the graft epicondyles have been resected to allow attachment of host epicondyles.

is used if the collateral ligaments are functioning; a greater degree of constraint is chosen if there are concerns about the stability to varus and valgus stress. We prefer to avoid hinged prostheses if at all possible, as we believe that the forces they create can contribute to a nonunion of the graft-host junction.

For femoral grafts, any residual host bone is then wrapped around the allograft and the step-cut junction. The junction may need further stabilization with an overlapping allograft cortical strut. Morcellized allograft and autograft is packed at the junction. In the rare situation in which a tibial graft requires supplemental fixation, longitudinal screws are placed medially and laterally. Cortical struts are not advisable on the tibial side as they make the construct bulky and could interfere with wound closure or cause tension on the skin.

Pitfalls

The first clinical decision to be made when treating a displaced periprosthetic fracture of the knee is whether to attempt to fix the fracture or manage it with revision TKA. Solid fixation is likely to be difficult to achieve in fractures that are directly adjacent to the femoral or tibial component. This is particularly true in elderly patients with osteoporotic bone and comminution. Furthermore, even if fixation is achieved in these fractures using modern devices such as locking plates, a period of postoperative immobilization is required. This can often lead to systemic complications associated with immobilization in the elderly as well as local problems, such as lost range of motion of the knee.

Similar to all revision TKA surgery, the principles of a successful reconstruction in this context include protection and preservation of the overlying skin. Because these injuries often result from a direct blow to the knee, one must be certain that the skin conditions are suitable for surgery. Ecchymotic, edematous skin should be given adequate time to improve before making surgical incisions through it.

Appropriate positioning of the joint line is of importance and may be difficult when the anatomy has been greatly distorted by previous TKA with superimposed bone loss and periprosthetic fracture. Landmarks such as the fibular head, medial epicondyle, or meniscal scar should be used to estimate the appropriate level for the joint. In addition, radiographs of the opposite, unaffected side can act as a guide to native joint line level.

Component malrotation is a common error in TKA surgery, and the difficulty of determining femoral and tibial rotation is compounded when landmarks are fractured or absent. The transepicondylar axis should be used if at all possible. When one of the epicondyles has been lost or fractured, a symmetric flexion gap at 90° of flexion may be used as a guide to correct femoral rotation. Ultimately, proper patellar tracking is the ultimate gauge of femoral rotation and should be assessed with trial implants in place, before cementing the definitive implant components.

Adequate reconstitution of bone loss and ligamentous insufficiency must be accomplished in the context of periprosthetic fracture. In particular, we have found that deficiency on the medial side that renders the MCL incompetent must be compensated for. Failure to either fix the medial condyle and restore MCL function or use a hinged prosthesis, which compensates for the MCL, will ultimately lead to catastrophic failure, with dislocation of the knee as a consequence (**Figure 7**).

Postoperative Regimen

The goal of rehabilitation after revision TKA surgery for periprosthetic fractures is rapid mobilization with immediate range-of-motion exercises and rapid progression to full weight bearing. In fact, this is one of the primary benefits of revision surgery over open reduction and internal fixation.

Our routine is to commence pharmacologic venous thromboembolism prophylaxis on the first postoperative day, using low-molecular-weight heparin injections. This is continued for a total of 10 to 14 days. First-generation cephalosporin prophylactic antibiotics are administered intravenously for 24 hours. Dressings and drains are removed at 48 hours postoperatively, and urinary catheters are discontinued within the first 2 days.

In all cases, stems are used, to obtain diaphyseal fit and augment implant fixation. Postoperative rehabilitation is commenced on the first postoperative day, including supervised range-of-motion exercise and mobilization, initially using a walker. Patients are progressively advanced from a walker to a cane as rapidly as possible. Quadriceps strengthening begins with extension over a roll and progresses to resisted exercises as tolerated. Active extension is restricted only in the rare cases in which a tibial tubercle osteotomy has been performed or a tibial tubercle fracture has been fixed. Patients are instructed to avoid active extension for 6 weeks in such circumstances.

When an AIC or structural allografts are used or large contained defects are filled with morcellized bone, weight bearing is restricted for 6 to 8 weeks. Weight bearing is then progressively advanced with the assistance of a physical therapist.

Results

The goals of treatment of periprosthetic fractures of the knee are to obtain and maintain good alignment, which provides stability and allows early range of motion.[4] Several options exist for the modern treatment of displaced periprosthetic fractures around a TKA, including retrograde intramedullary nails, blade plates, condylar buttress plates, and locked condylar plates. Early studies using plates and screws showed a high incidence of fixation failure and other complications,[15-18] but modern techniques and implants have been more successful. However, results for very distal femoral fractures, particularly when combined with osteoporotic bone, have been less satisfactory. After reviewing a series of 21 fractures above well-fixed femoral components fixed with

FIGURE 7

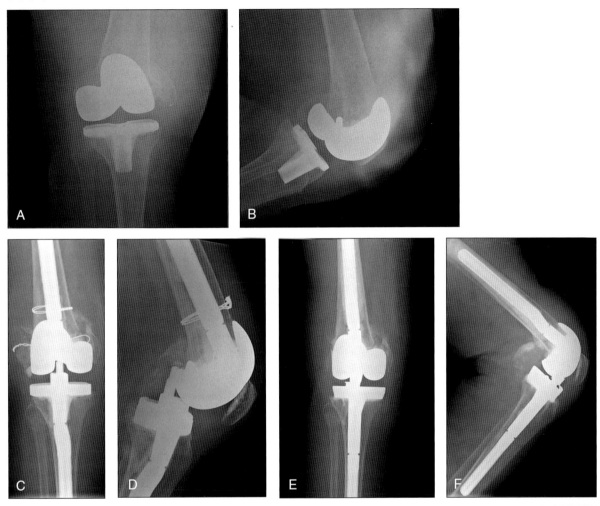

AP (**A**) and lateral (**B**) radiographs of a distal femoral periprosthetic fracture with intercondylar split. **C**, Postoperative AP view obtained after revision total knee arthroplasty with a semiconstrained prosthesis. **D**, Cross-table lateral view demonstrates dislocation of semiconstrained revision total knee arthroplasty. AP (**E**) and lateral (**F**) radiographs obtained after revision to a hinged total knee prosthesis.

indirect reduction and plates, Kolb et al[19] suggested that such fracture fixation techniques are best used in proximal fractures with minimal comminution and in the hands of experienced trauma surgeons. In a meta-analysis of 195 such fractures, Chen et al[20] found superior results in displaced fractures that were treated with revision in comparison to those treated with open reduction and internal fixation. Bezwada et al[21] conducted a

retrospective review of 30 displaced supracondylar femoral periprosthetic fractures, 18 of which were treated with retrograde intramedullary nails and 12 of which were treated with open reduction and internal fixation using distal femoral periarticular plates. The authors considered the outcomes of these two treatment methods to be successful. It is worth noting, however, that the average time to union of 10 weeks (range, 4 to

16 weeks) necessitated a prolonged period of protected weight bearing. Additionally, in this series of 30 fractures, there was 1 varus nonunion, 1 amputation for sepsis, and 13 knees that united in 5° or more of valgus. This series seems to indicate that intramedullary nail or plate fixation may provide a high rate of union but ideal alignment may be difficult to achieve. This is likely to be even more relevant in very distal fractures in osteoporotic bone.

Use of modern distal femoral replacement prostheses specifically for periprosthetic fractures of the knee is not well reported in the literature. Jones et al[22] reported on the use of the S-ROM mobile-bearing hinge total knee replacement (DePuy Orthopaedics, Warsaw, IN), which has modular sleeves to allow fill of metaphyseal and diaphyseal defects. Although none of the 16 knees in this series had surgery for periprosthetic fracture, all had ligamentous instability, bone loss, or both. At a minimum of 2 years' follow-up, significant improvements in pain, motion, and stability were noted and there was no evidence of loosening, and complete bone apposition occurred in all but 1 case. In the oncology literature, the 5-year survivorship of such bone-replacing implants in the context of tumor resection is 80% to 90%.[23,24] Pour et al[25] reported a survival rate of 79.6% at 1 year and 68.2% at 5 years with the use of the Kinematic rotating-hinge knee implant (Stryker Orthopaedics, Mahwah, NJ) or the Finn rotating-hinge prosthesis (Biomet, Warsaw, IN) in 44 cases, including 4 periprosthetic fractures, with a mean follow-up of 4.2 years (range, 2.0 to 8.0 years). Springer et al[26] reported on a series of 26 knees, including 12 periprosthetic fractures, treated with a modular segmental distal femoral–replacing rotating-hinge prosthesis and noted improvement in Knee Society knee and functional scores at a mean follow-up of 58.5 months. Complications occurred in eight patients, with infection being most common (five patients).

Conclusions

Management of periprosthetic fractures of the knee is challenging, particularly when the fracture is immediately adjacent to implants, because of compromised bone stock, frequent loss of ligamentous attachments, and an elderly group of patients who poorly tolerate prolonged immobility. The goals of surgery for these fractures are to restore the limb's structural ability to bear weight and the ligamentous integrity and range of motion of the knee. For fractures that are immediately adjacent to the femoral or tibial implant, particularly when associated with poor bone quality or a loose implant, revision TKA is preferable to attempted plate osteosynthesis. In most cases, typical principles of revision TKA surgery apply, including the use of augments and bone grafts for restitution of bone loss. In certain cases of extreme bone deficiency, bone replacement megaprostheses may be required. Regardless of the technique chosen, these procedures are complex and require considerable experience and resources.

References

1. Jeong GK, Pettrone SK, Liporace FA, Meere PA: "Floating total knee": Ipsilateral periprosthetic fractures of the distal femur and proximal tibia after total knee arthroplasty. *J Arthroplasty* 2006;21(1):138-140.

2. Kurtz S, Mowat F, Ong K, Chan N, Lau E, Halpern M: Prevalence of primary and revision total hip and knee arthroplasty in the United States from 1990 through 2002. *J Bone Joint Surg Am* 2005;87(7):1487-1497.

3. Fujii R, Ueda T, Tamai N, Myoui A, Yoshikawa H: Salvage surgery for persistent femoral nonunion after total knee arthroplasty using a megaprosthesis. *J Orthop Sci* 2006;11(4):401-404.

4. Dennis DA: Periprosthetic fractures following total knee arthroplasty. *Instr Course Lect* 2001;50:379-389.

5. Alden KJ, Duncan WH, Trousdale RT, Pagnano MW, Haidukewych GJ: Intraoperative fracture during primary total knee arthroplasty. *Clin Orthop Relat Res* 2010;468(1):90-95.

6. Gross AE: Periprosthetic fractures of the knee: Puzzle pieces. *J Arthroplasty* 2004;19(4, Suppl 1):47-50.

7. Zalzal P, Backstein D, Gross AE, Papini M: Notching of the anterior femoral cortex during total knee arthroplasty characteristics that increase local stresses. *J Arthroplasty* 2006;21(5):737-743.

8. Hirsch DM, Bhalla S, Roffman M: Supracondylar fracture of the femur following total knee replacement: Report of four cases. *J Bone Joint Surg Am* 1981;63A:162-163.

9. Bogoch E, Hastings D, Gross A, Gschwend N: Supracondylar fractures of the femur adjacent to resurfacing and MacIntosh arthroplasties of the knee in patients with rheumatoid arthritis. *Clin Orthop Relat Res* 1988;229:213-220.

10. Lombardi AV Jr, Mallory TH, Waterman RA, Eberle RW: Intercondylar distal femoral fracture: An unreported complication of posterior-stabilized total knee arthroplasty. *J Arthroplasty* 1995;10(5):643-650.

11. Larson JE, Chao EY, Fitzgerald RH: Bypassing femoral cortical defects with cemented intramedullary stems. *J Orthop Res* 1991;9(3):414-421.

12. Culp RW, Schmidt RG, Hanks G, Mak A, Esterhai JL Jr, Heppenstall RB: Supracondylar fracture of the femur following prosthetic knee arthroplasty. *Clin Orthop Relat Res* 1987;222:212-222.

13. Parvizi J, Jain N, Schmidt AH: Periprosthetic knee fractures. *J Orthop Trauma* 2008;22(9):663-671.

14. Backstein D, Safir O, Gross A: Periprosthetic fractures of the knee. *J Arthroplasty* 2007;22(4, Suppl 1):45-49.

15. Moran MC, Brick GW, Sledge CB, Dysart SH, Chien EP: Supracondylar femoral fracture following total knee arthroplasty. *Clin Orthop Relat Res* 1996;324:196-209.

16. Figgie MP, Goldberg VM, Figgie HE III, Sobel M: The results of treatment of supracondylar fracture above total knee arthroplasty. *J Arthroplasty* 1990;5(3):267-276.

17. Cordeiro EN, Costa RC, Carazzato JG, Silva JdosS: Periprosthetic fractures in patients with total knee arthroplasties. *Clin Orthop Relat Res* 1990;252:182-189.

18. Nielsen BF, Petersen VS, Varmarken JE: Fracture of the femur after knee arthroplasty. *Acta Orthop Scand* 1988;59(2):155-157.

19. Kolb K, Koller H, Lorenz I, et al: Operative treatment of distal femoral fractures above total knee arthroplasty with the indirect reduction technique: A long-term follow-up study. *Injury* 2009;40(4):433-439.

20. Chen F, Mont MA, Bachner RS: Management of ipsilateral supracondylar femur fractures following total knee arthroplasty. *J Arthroplasty* 1994;9(5):521-526.

21. Bezwada HP, Neubauer P, Baker J, Israelite CL, Johanson NA: Periprosthetic supracondylar femur fractures following total knee arthroplasty. *J Arthroplasty* 2004;19(4):453-458.

22. Jones RE, Skedros JG, Chan AJ, Beauchamp DH, Harkins PC: Total knee arthroplasty using the S-ROM mobile-bearing hinge prosthesis. *J Arthroplasty* 2001;16(3):279-287.

23. Choong PF, Sim FH, Pritchard DJ, Rock MG, Chao EY: Megaprostheses after resection of distal femoral tumors: A rotating hinge design in 30 patients followed for 2-7 years. *Acta Orthop Scand* 1996;67(4):345-351.

24. Mittermayer F, Krepler P, Dominkus M, et al: Long-term followup of uncemented tumor endoprostheses for the lower extremity. *Clin Orthop Relat Res* 2001;388:167-177.

25. Pour AE, Parvizi J, Slenker N, Purtill JJ, Sharkey PF: Rotating hinged total knee replacement: Use with caution. *J Bone Joint Surg Am* 2007;89(8):1735-1741.

26. Springer BD, Sim FH, Hanssen AD, Lewallen DG: The modular segmental kinematic rotating hinge for non-neoplastic limb salvage. *Clin Orthop Relat Res* 2004;421:181-187.

Revision Total Knee Arthroplasty for Instability

Gregg R. Klein, MD
Harlan B. Levine, MD

Introduction

The long-term success of total knee arthroplasty (TKA) has been well documented, but failures do occur. Revisions performed for unstable TKAs account for approximately 20% of revision TKAs performed.[1-3] Sharkey et al[2] reviewed the reasons for failure in 212 knee revisions and found that instability was the third most common cause of failure.

Four types of instability may occur following TKA: (1) axial (also called extension or varus/valgus) instability; (2) recurvatum (hyperextension); (3) anterior-posterior (flexion) instability; and (4) global instability.

The goal of management of the unstable knee is to correct the predisposing factor(s) responsible for the instability. Treatment options include soft-tissue procedures, polyethylene liner exchange, and revision TKA. To correct instability in a TKA, revision of the components is often necessary to balance the flexion and extension gaps and appropriately tension the soft tissues. When gap balancing or soft-tissue balancing proves to be unattainable, constrained revision implants are necessary. Different levels of component constraint include standard cruciate-retaining (CR) implants, CR implants that are ultracongruent, posterior-stabilized (PS) implants, PS-plus implants, varus/valgus constrained implants, and hinged components.[4] The minimum amount of constraint that is necessary to achieve a well-balanced knee should be used, as increasing constraint causes load transmission to the prosthesis–host bone interfaces that may increase rates of loosening.

Diagnosis

The diagnosis may be obvious, as in gross ligamentous incompetence, or it may be subtle, as in mild flexion instability manifesting as recurrent effusions and diffuse pain. It is important to try to obtain information regarding the reason for the original TKA, the presence of initial deformity (severe varus, valgus, recurvatum, or flexion contractures), previous procedures, surgical approach and ligaments released, and the type of prosthesis used (CR versus cruciate-substituting). Patients with severe deformity often require aggressive ligamentous releases. At the original surgery, these releases may have been inadequate, resulting in recurrent varus/valgus loads or deformity, or they may have been overaggressive, resulting in subtle ligamentous imbalance. The timing of the instability is important as well. Instability symptoms that occur early after the index procedure may be a consequence of technical errors. Symptoms that occur late may be due to posterior cruciate ligament (PCL) rupture, polyethylene wear, or component loosening. The effects and clinical symptoms of instability

Dr. Klein or an immediate family member serves as a board member, owner, officer, or committee member of Surgicare Surgical Associates of Carlstadt, LLC; is a member of a speakers' bureau or has made paid presentations on behalf of Zimmer; serves as a paid consultant to or is an employee of Biomet and Zimmer; and has received research or institutional support from Zimmer. Dr. Levine or an immediate family member serves as a paid consultant to or is an employee of Biomet and has received research or institutional support from Zimmer.

are compounded by malalignment.[5] In a well-aligned knee, small amounts of laxity or instability may be tolerated; however, as malalignment occurs, relatively small amounts of laxity may be magnified by improper component alignment or position. A history of trauma should be questioned as well. Patients should be asked if there were any specific events or circumstances that led to an acute change in their condition. Late PCL rupture may occur in a previously well-functioning knee.[6]

Intrinsic patient-related factors may be related to unstable knee replacements. Patients with a history of neuromuscular disease (eg, poliomyelitis, multiple sclerosis), collagen vascular diseases (eg, Ehler-Danlos syndrome), rheumatoid arthritis, or significant weight loss such as after gastric bypass[7] have a higher risk of instability after primary TKA. Ipsilateral or contralateral hip, knee, and ankle deformities may cause gait abnormalities and may result in inadequate alignment and instability at the knee. Gait abnormalities, quadriceps weakness, and/or weak hip abductors may have caused the initial deformity and may result in premature failure of the replaced knee.[8] If these are not corrected, revision TKA will fail as well.[3] TKA in the obese patient has been associated with difficulty in exposure and possible avulsion of the medial collateral ligament (MCL), leading to postoperative instability.[9]

A patient with instability of a TKA may have symptoms ranging from subtle pain and tenderness to gross instability or history of dislocation. It is important to distinguish tibial/femoral instability from patellofemoral instability, as patients often confuse these. Symptoms of tibial/femoral instability include anterior knee pain, recurrent swelling, and giving way.[1,10] Some patients report that they have difficulty "getting their knee in gear";[1] others report that the knee is always swollen, or feels "full." The swelling is often activity related but does not completely resolve with rest. The patient often reports difficulty in ascending or descending stairs. Either diffuse or localized pain may be present. Some patients have symptoms isolated to the anterior medial knee over the pes anserinus and retinaculum.[11]

An accurate and thorough physical examination is essential.[6,11] Range of motion of an unstable knee is generally good to excellent. Patients will often relate a history of an easy postoperative recovery, with early restoration of motion without difficulty. The knee should be evaluated for varus/valgus instability in full extension, in 30° of flexion, and in 90° of flexion. In full extension, the posterior capsule is tight and may give a false sense of collateral ligament tightness. At 30° of flexion, the posterior capsule and posterior structures are lax, and collateral ligament laxity may be unmasked.

At 90° of flexion, varus/valgus laxity may be appreciated, but the addition of hip motion makes the examination more difficult. At 90° of flexion, anterior-posterior stability should be examined. This is best performed with the patient sitting and the knee flexed 90°, hanging over the edge of the examination table. An anterior and posterior drawer test may be applied. It is important to compare the results with the contralateral knee, as variable amounts of laxity may be present from patient to patient. For CR knees, the examiner should examine the PCL and look for posterior sag, and a quadriceps active test should be performed. In the quadriceps active test, the flexed knee reveals a reduction of the tibia from its posteriorly subluxated position to the neutral position as the quadriceps is fired. On radiographs, implants often appear well-aligned on the AP view, but posterior subluxation of the tibia under the femur may be seen on the lateral view.[12]

Prior to revision surgery, a preoperative aspiration should be performed to rule out infection. This may also help to confirm the diagnosis of instability. A bloody effusion may suggest joint instability. Fehring and Valadie[1] reported a predominance of red blood cells (mean, 64,000/mm[3]) in knees that were aspirated before being revised for instability.

AXIAL INSTABILITY

Axial instability may be the result of ligamentous imbalance, axial malalignment, eccentric polyethylene wear, implant failure, excessive bony resection, component malposition, subsidence or loosening, or gross ligamentous failure (**Table 1**). Axial instability may be further classified as either symmetric or asymmetric.[13,14]

Symmetric axial instability occurs when the extension gap is not completely filled by the prosthetic components. This is usually the result of excessive bone resection and may occur on both the femoral and tibial sides. If the tibial resection is too large, the flexion and extension gaps will be equally affected. This may be corrected by using a thicker polyethylene insert or using modular augments below the tibial tray. Because the

TABLE 1 **Causes of Axial Instability**

Excessive bony resection
Inadequate ligament releases
Overaggressive ligament releases
Iatrogenic ligament injury
Subsidence or loosening
Polyethylene wear
Axial malalignment
Component malposition
Implant failure

FIGURE 1

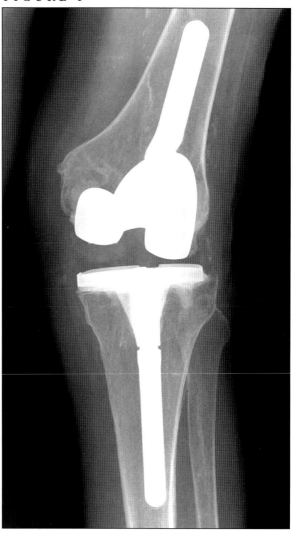

AP radiograph demonstrates gross medial collateral ligament incompetence.

flexion and extension gaps are equally affected, the function of the knee should not be compromised. Excessive distal femoral resection is more difficult to correct. Overaggressive resection of distal femoral bone will leave a larger extension gap than flexion gap. Simply using a bigger polyethylene articular surface to fill the extension gap will result in an overly tight flexion gap that will limit knee flexion and elevate the joint line, which will cause patella infera that may also limit knee flexion and cause anterior knee pain. In a CR knee, joint-line elevation also may cause improper balance of the PCL and thus should be avoided. In such cases, to reduce the relative size of the extension gap, augments should be placed on the distal femur to achieve symmetry between the extension and flexion gaps. Such modular augments are readily available in most revision knee systems today.

Asymmetric extension instability occurs more commonly than symmetric instability. It may be the result of malalignment of the bone cuts, bone loss, subsidence, aseptic loosening, collateral ligament imbalance, or gross ligamentous failure. Collateral ligament imbalance may be caused by either underrelease or overrelease of the preoperative deformity or by traumatic ligamentous disruption (**Figure 1**). Of these, undercorrection of the deformity and failure to obtain a balanced extension gap is the most common cause for asymmetric instability (**Figure 2**). This often occurs intraoperatively, when the surgeon is concerned about overreleasing and limits the surgical releases to avoid "doing too much."[13] This may occur with both varus and valgus knees. A varus knee that is undercorrected, particularly if it is also left in an overall varus alignment, may fail in varus.

Overcorrection or direct ligament injury may occur on rare occasions. This may be corrected by direct liga-mentous repair[15] and/or the use of a more constrained implant. Undercorrection of a valgus knee will leave the medial soft tissues lax. Over time, the valgus deformity may recur and potentially need to be revised.

In contrast, Koo and Choi[16] recently reported on a series of 15 varus knees that were complicated by complete detachment of the MCL from the tibial insertion.

FIGURE 2

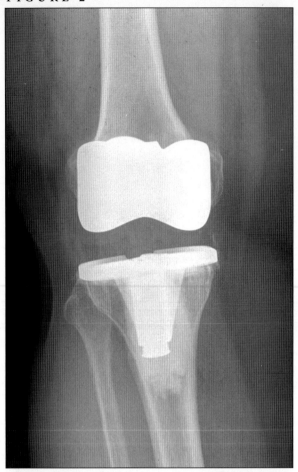

AP radiograph of a knee in which the medial structures were under-released demonstrates unbalanced medial and lateral gaps in extension. Note the overall varus alignment of the knee.

These knees were treated by increasing the articular insert size to obtain balanced gaps. Braces or immobilization was not used. No clinical instability or complications had developed at a minimum of 2 years postoperatively. Specific techniques for valgus and varus correction are beyond the scope of this chapter.

RECURVATUM

Recurvatum, or hyperextension, after TKA is rare. When it does occur, it is most commonly seen in patients with neuromuscular diseases such as poliomyelitis, spinal stenosis, or multiple sclerosis.[17,18] Patients with such conditions may have poor ipsilateral extremity strength. Such weakness, especially in the quadriceps, forces these patients to hyperextend the knee and lock it during stance phase to prevent the knee from collapsing into flexion. This repetitive hyperextension torque may result in attenuation or stretching of the posterior capsule (**Figure 3**). TKA in these patients should be performed with caution. Removing the ability to hyperextend the knee may limit the patient's ability to lock the knee in extension during stance phase and therefore limit the ability to walk. However, allowing the patient to hyperextend after TKA risks stretching the posterior capsule and recurrence of the deformity. When performing TKA in patients at risk for recurvatum deformity, a smaller distal femoral resection may be performed to create a smaller extension gap. Alternatively, distal femoral augments may be used to lessen the size of the extension gap. In cases of preoperative recurvatum in patients with neuromuscular disorders, the knee may be left with a slight flexion contracture intraoperatively to allow for some stretching of the posterior capsule postoperatively. However, this may make walking difficult for these patients, as leaving them with a flexion contracture may limit their ability to lock out the knee during stance phase. Krackow and Weiss[17] have described a method of surgically translating the collateral ligament origins to physiologically account for the hyperextension deformity.

The use of linked rotating-hinge implants for the treatment of recurvatum in the setting of neuromuscular disorders has been gaining popularity. Giori and Lewallen[19] reported on 16 knees in patients with poliomyelitis who had undergone TKA and found better results and function in patients with at least antigravity abduction strength preoperatively. Patients with poor quadriceps function who have less than antigravity strength treated with conventional TKA showed poor pain relief, recurrence of hyperextension, and ligamentous laxity. The authors suggested fusion or the use of a hinged knee component in these patients.[19]

FLEXION INSTABILITY

Flexion instability is imbalance in the flexion gap or a flexion gap that is larger than the extension gap. Causes of flexion instability are listed in **Table 2**. Flexion insta-

FIGURE 3

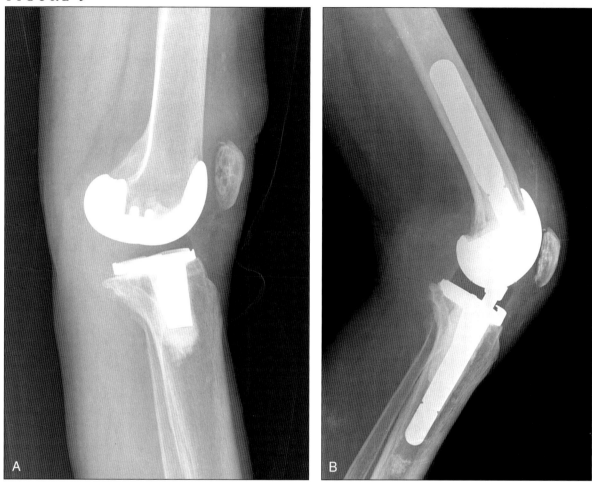

Radiographs of a patient with multiple sclerosis who was treated with a total knee arthroplasty. Progressive recurvatum developed postoperatively. **A**, Lateral radiograph demonstrates the recurvatum. **B**, Lateral radiograph obtained after revision to a hinged construct with a hyperextension stop.

bility may have various presentations, from vague reports of pain and swelling to gross tibiofemoral dislocation. Approximately 5 mm of anterior-posterior translation is needed for physiologic range of motion.[20] Anterior-posterior translation greater than 5 mm can result in symptoms related to instability. Flexion instability may occur in many different scenarios, some of which are related to surgical technique. Often the radiographs reveal a well-aligned and well-positioned TKA. The diag-

nosis is often made by a detailed history and physical examination, and it may be confirmed with stress radiographs.

A large flexion gap may be caused by inadequate implant size or improper femoral component position. During a TKA, placing the femoral cutting block too anterior on the distal femur will result in an excessive posterior condylar resection, causing a larger flexion gap than extension gap. Similarly, undersizing the

TABLE 2 Causes of Flexion Instability

Anterior placement of the femur
Undersized femoral component
Excessive tibial slope
Mismanagement of flexion contracture
Malrotation of femoral component
Undersized femoral component used to match bone defects in revision TKA
Spine/cam properties
Excessive release in valgus knee
Inadequate balance of PCL
Late rupture of PCL
Rheumatoid arthritis/collagen vascular disease
Polyethylene wear
PCL = posterior cruciate ligament, TKA = total knee arthroplasty.

femoral component (**Figure 4**) will also result in an excessive posterior condylar resection and resulting mismatch between the flexion and extension gaps. Placement of an articular insert that fills the flexion gap will result in a tight extension gap; therefore, a postoperative flexion contracture will occur. To correct the flexion contracture, the knee may be balanced by a posterior capsular release and/or resecting additional distal femur and placing the femoral component more proximally. Although resecting additional distal femoral bone will obtain balanced gaps, it also will elevate the joint line, causing patella infera, and in CR knees it may cause ligamentous imbalance of the PCL.

Over the years, implant manufacturers have released a broader range of femoral implant sizes, allowing for improved gap balancing.[21] Gap balancing errors still occur today, especially when femoral sizing is based on the medial-lateral dimensions of the implants. In some patients, particularly women, the femur has a relatively narrower medial-lateral dimension compared to the anterior-posterior dimension. For such patients, a femoral implant that is sized to the relatively narrow medial-lateral dimensions of the distal femur will be undersized in the anterior-posterior plane and therefore create a larger flexion gap than extension gap. Some implants have been designed with medial-lateral dimensions that are smaller relative to the anterior-posterior dimensions

to allow for better gap balancing without creating component overhang medially and/or laterally.

Anterior placement of the femoral component can be avoided by using a posterior referencing system and critically evaluating the amount of posterior condylar resection before posterior condylar osteotomy. A posterior referencing system allows a predictive posterior condylar resection. However, risks of anterior femoral notching or anterior compartment overstuffing occur, and the anterior cut should be evaluated before actually completing the resection. If the amount of posterior condylar bone that is to be removed is excessive, the femoral cutting block may need to be moved posteriorly or the femoral component upsized.

In revision TKA, a common error is to size the femoral component based on remaining distal femoral bone (**Figure 5**). This often results in undersizing the femoral component and creates an overly large flexion gap. To avoid this error in the revision setting, it is often necessary to size the femoral component independently of the remaining host bone and then substitute for bony defects in the posterior condyles with modular augments. Another technique used to fill the flexion gap is to posteriorize the femoral component using an offset femoral stem (**Figure 6**). This use of offset stems allows the femoral component to be placed more posterior relative to the femoral shaft, which will also lessen the flexion gap.

On the tibial side, excessive slope in the proximal tibial osteotomy alone or in combination with a tibial component that already has slope built into it will cause flexion instability. In primary TKA, it is important to understand the knee system and tibial component that is being used to create the appropriate slope in the proximal tibial osteotomy. Manufacturers of TKA implants all have different specifications and different recommended amounts of posterior slope. In evaluating radiographs for clues of potential flexion instability, it is important to critically evaluate the tibial slope (**Figure 7**). In general, PS knees tend to have less tibial slope than CR knees. However, excessive posterior slope or excessive tibial resection in a CR knee should raise suspicion about the integrity of the PCL if the cut is below the PCL insertion.

In the revision situation, the use of an intramedullary cutting device and intramedullary stems allows for the

FIGURE 4

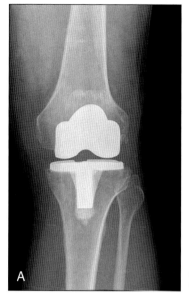 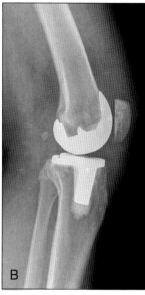 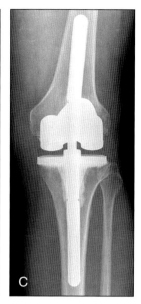 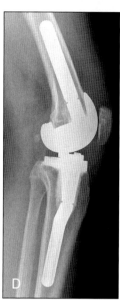

AP (**A**) and lateral (**B**) radiographs of a knee after total knee arthroplasty with an undersized femoral component that resulted in postoperative flexion instability. AP (**C**) and lateral (**D**) radiographs show the knee after revision to a larger femoral component with posterior condylar augments to balance the flexion space.

creation of neutral tibial slope. Most revision systems have the necessary tibial slope built into the revision implants to allow for normal knee kinematics. Inadequate management of a preoperative flexion contracture will often lead to flexion instability. If a substantial preoperative flexion contracture exists, the knee will likely be tighter in extension than flexion. The tendency is to use a smaller polyethylene insert to obtain full extension. This will effectively result in inadequate filling of the flexion gap and thus flexion instability. Flexion contractures should be managed in the classic manner, including resection of posterior osteophytes, a posterior capsule release, and then, if necessary, resection of additional distal femoral bone to achieve full extension.

Malrotation of the femoral component will also lead to imbalance of the flexion gap. Relative internal rotation of the femoral component will lead to a larger lateral flexion gap, while relative external rotation of the femoral implant will lead to a larger medial flexion gap and subsequent instability.[20] Such instability is best treated by prevention of malrotation of the femoral component.

Classic landmarks used to define appropriate femoral rotation, such as the AP axis of the femur[22] and epicondylar axis,[23] should be used to ensure proper component orientation. The use of the posterior condylar axis to define femoral rotation should be avoided in the following situations: (1) large valgus deformities, in which relative hypoplasia of the lateral femoral condyle may be present, creating internal rotation of the femoral implant; (2) severe varus deformities, in which excessive wear of the medial femoral condyle may be present, resulting in excessive femoral component external rotation; or (3) revisions with deficient posterior bone. Some surgeons use tensioning devices to evaluate ligament balance to create symmetric medial and lateral flexion gaps and achieve femoral rotation parallel to the tibial surface.

Polyethylene wear is another cause of flexion instability. This is most pronounced when eccentric wear of the posterior tibial polyethylene is present. This usually occurs late, after a TKA has been functioning well for years. If the wear is posterior on the polyethylene, it may be difficult to appreciate on standard radiographs.

FIGURE 5

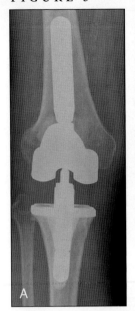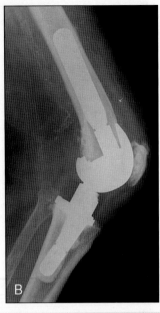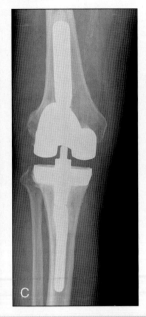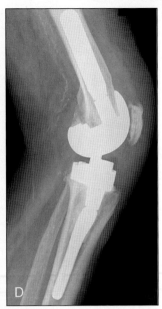

AP (**A**) and lateral (**B**) radiographs of a knee after revision total knee arthroplasty with an undersized femoral component. At the time of revision, the femoral component was sized based on the remaining bone stock available. Note the large polyethylene articular surface used to fill the flexion gap, which resulted in raising the joint line. AP (**C**) and lateral (**D**) radiographs after rerevision. The femoral component was increased two sizes, which allowed for a smaller articular surface to balance the flexion space.

Isolated revision of the polyethylene insert should be used with caution and reserved for well-aligned knees with stable prosthesis–host bone interfaces that present with late polyethylene wear.

Some forms of flexion instability are unique to the prosthesis being evaluated with respect to PCL-retaining and PCL-substituting designs. In CR knees, the functional status of the PCL is essential. Early failure of CR implants is often due to inadequate balancing of the PCL. Both underrelease and overrelease of the PCL may cause flexion instability. When the PCL is overreleased, the biomechanics of the knee are altered and there may even be paradoxical anterior femoral translation of the femur on the tibia in flexion and resultant flexion instability. In addition, overrelease or complete release may result in a larger flexion gap and flexion instability as described above. Underrelease of the PCL may lead to stiffness and a tight flexion gap and premature polyethylene wear. Patients may report a period of good function followed by an "event" and then symptoms of instability. This is often a sign of late rupture of the PCL.[24]

The results of nonsurgical treatment of flexion instability in CR knees are poor. In addition, isolated polyethylene revision has led to poor outcomes in this population.[25,26] Pagnano et al[11] and Waslewski et al[6] have reported poor results with isolated polyethylene exchange in CR implants. Most patients are ideally treated with a revision of the components to a PS design and vigilant flexion/extension gap balancing.[11]

Laskin and O'Flynn[27] reported on a series of patients with rheumatoid arthritis in whom recurvatum and flexion instability developed. They found an increased incidence of instability and recurvatum in CR knees compared with PS knees. This is likely related to the inherent properties of the tissues in patients with rheumatoid arthritis.[27] In contrast, Archibeck et al[28] reported satisfactory results in patients with rheumatoid arthritis treated with CR TKAs. The authors identified

FIGURE 6

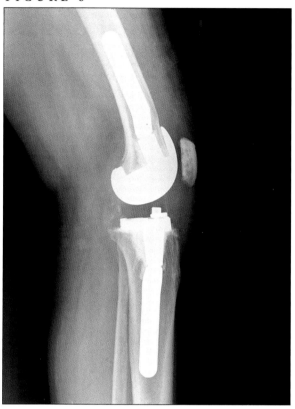

Lateral radiograph of a knee after revision total knee arthroplasty shows an offset femoral stem that posteriorizes the femoral component relative to the femoral canal. This effectively reduces the flexion space.

FIGURE 7

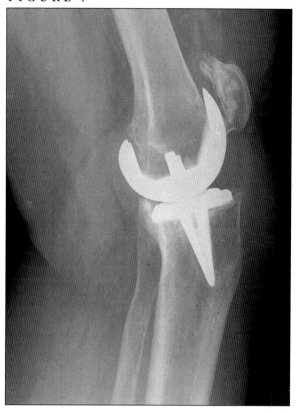

Lateral radiograph of a knee obtained after total knee arthroplasty demonstrates excessive slope of the tibial component, which resulted in postoperative flexion instability.

posterior instability in only 2 (2.8%) of the 72 knees followed at a mean of 10.5 years.

Flexion instability may develop in knees with PS implants, based on the properties and design of the implants. Each PS design has its own cam/post relationship that may inherently predispose to instability or gross dislocation. Certain height or positional characteristics of the tibial post have been shown to predispose to frank tibial-femoral dislocation.[29] Historically, acute dislocation after a PS TKA occurred in approximately 1% to 2% of knees.[21] The dislocation rate has been dramatically decreased over the years by improvements and changes in the post/cam designs.[30] For example, the Insall-Burstein II prosthesis elevated and anteriorly translated the post 2 mm, compared with the Insall-Burstein I design. This design change reduced the dislocation rate from 2.5% to 0.2%.[21,31] The mechanism of posterior dislocation[29,31,32] of the tibia on the femur is usually associated with deep knee flexion and a varus force (ie, figure-of-4 position). Dislocations generally need to be reduced under anesthesia or sedation followed by 3 to 4 weeks of immobilization in extension in a cast or brace. In one series, two thirds of knees treated with this protocol were successful and did not require additional surgery.[31] If surgical intervention is necessary, revision to a larger articular insert may be successful if balanced flexion and extension gaps can be obtained. If balanced gaps are not possible, revision to a larger femoral component or a more constrained construct may be necessary.

Knees that have obtained flexion quickly in the postoperative period are at higher risk for dislocation in a PS design.[31] Theoretically, these knees are less tight, may be poorly balanced and potentially unstable, and thus exhibit early instability, allowing early flexion. If frank instability develops, revision arthroplasty is usually necessary. Proposed mechanisms of dislocation include patients with hamstring contractures combined with a posteriorly directed force. Other mechanisms include figure-of-4 positioning in knees that are rotationally unstable.

Occasionally, the post of the articular surface on a PS TKA may fracture and late flexion instability may develop. If late-onset sagittal plane instability develops and posterior sag is present, severe post wear or fracture should be suspected. This may be managed with revision of the polyethylene articular surface. However, before such isolated articular surface revision, an attempt should be made to identify and correct any potential source of abnormally large stresses at the tibial post/femoral cam junction. Finally, patients with PS knees who had a preoperative valgus deformity requiring extensive valgus releases are at risk for flexion instability and even dislocation of the knee.[33] In such knees, a rotatory dislocation may occur as knee flexion is combined with a varus force that is unable to be controlled by the released lateral soft tissues. Few reports have been published focusing on revision TKA for flexion instability in PS implants. Schwab et al[10] reported on 10 patients with flexion instability without dislocation in PS knees. In this cohort, patients reported a sense of instability without giving way, difficulty with stairs, recurrent effusions, and diffuse anterior knee pain. Examination revealed substantial anterior translation, effusions, and soft-tissue tenderness in multiple areas, including the pes anserinus, peripatellar tissues, and hamstrings. Various revision techniques were used, including isolated polyethylene exchange in 2 patients and full revision in 8 patients, with upsizing of the femur in 7 of the 8. The revision procedures were reliable in relieving pain, and stability was improved in 9 of 10 patients.[10]

Global Instability

Global instability is a combination of the various types of instability listed above, including a combination of flexion and extension instability with or without recurvatum. All the causes for the other forms of instability may result in an unstable knee in multiple directions. Often soft-tissue compromise or collagen vascular diseases manifest with global instability. Treatment is aimed at correction of the underlying cause of instability, and constrained or hinged implants may be necessary. Global instability can develop in patients with extensor mechanism dysfunction, as these patients compensate for the weak extensor mechanism by a back-legged gait that may result in a recurvatum or global instability pattern.[12] More recently, it has been reported that the risk of instability developing in an otherwise well-functioning knee is higher in patients who have a gastric bypass after TKA.[7]

References

1. Fehring TK, Valadie AL: Knee instability after total knee arthroplasty. *Clin Orthop Relat Res* 1994;299:157-162.

2. Sharkey PF, Hozack WJ, Rothman RH, Shastri S, Jacoby SM: Insall Award paper: Why are total knee arthroplasties failing today? *Clin Orthop Relat Res* 2002;404:7-13.

3. Vince KG: Why knees fail. *J Arthroplasty* 2003;18(3, Suppl 1)39-44.

4. Rorabeck CH: Managing instability following total knee replacement. *Orthopedics* 2001;24(9):903-904.

5. Moreland JR: Mechanisms of failure in total knee arthroplasty. *Clin Orthop Relat Res* 1988;226:49-64.

6. Waslewski GL, Marson BM, Benjamin JB: Early, incapacitating instability of posterior cruciate ligament-retaining total knee arthroplasty. *J Arthroplasty* 1998;13(7):763-767.

7. Bezwada H, Nazarian DG, Booth RE Jr: Abstract: Instability in TKA following bariatric surgery. *2009 Annual Meeting Proceedings.* Rosemont, IL, American Academy of Orthopaedic Surgeons, 2009, p 525.

8. Vince KG, Abdeen A, Sugimori T: The unstable total knee arthroplasty: Causes and cures. *J Arthroplasty* 2006;21(4, Suppl 1)44-49.

9. Winiarsky R, Barth P, Lotke P: Total knee arthroplasty in morbidly obese patients. *J Bone Joint Surg Am* 1998;80(12):1770-1774.

10. Schwab JH, Haidukewych GJ, Hanssen AD, Jacofsky DJ, Pagnano MW: Flexion instability without dislocation after posterior stabilized total knees. *Clin Orthop Relat Res* 2005;440:96-100.

11. Pagnano MW, Hanssen AD, Lewallen DG, Stuart MJ: Flexion instability after primary posterior cruciate retaining total knee arthroplasty. *Clin Orthop Relat Res* 1998;356:39-46.

12. McAuley JP, Engh GA, Ammeen DJ: Treatment of the unstable total knee arthroplasty. *Instr Course Lect* 2004;53:237-241.

13. Kelly MA: Ligament instability in total knee arthroplasty. *Instr Course Lect* 2001;50:399-401.

14. Parratte S, Pagnano MW: Instability after total knee arthroplasty. *J Bone Joint Surg Am* 2008;90(1):184-194.

15. Krackow KA, Jones MM, Teeny SM, Hungerford DS: Primary total knee arthroplasty in patients with fixed valgus deformity. *Clin Orthop Relat Res* 1991;273:9-18.

16. Koo MH, Choi CH: Conservative treatment for the intraoperative detachment of medial collateral ligament from the tibial attachment site during primary total knee arthroplasty. *J Arthroplasty* 2009;24(8):1249-1253.

17. Krackow KA, Weiss AP: Recurvatum deformity complicating performance of total knee arthroplasty: A brief note. *J Bone Joint Surg Am* 1990;72(2):268-271.

18. Meding JB, Keating EM, Ritter MA, Faris PM, Berend ME: Genu recurvatum in total knee replacement. *Clin Orthop Relat Res* 2003;416:64-67.

19. Giori NJ, Lewallen DG: Total knee arthroplasty in limbs affected by poliomyelitis. *J Bone Joint Surg Am* 2002; 84-A(7):1157-1161.

20. Warren PJ, Olanlokun TK, Cobb AG, Walker PS, Iverson BF: Laxity and function in knee replacements: A comparative study of three prosthetic designs. *Clin Orthop Relat Res* 1994;305:200-208.

21. Clarke HD, Scuderi GR: Flexion instability in primary total knee replacement. *J Knee Surg* 2003;16(2):123-128.

22. Whiteside LA, Arima J: The anteroposterior axis for femoral rotational alignment in valgus total knee arthroplasty. *Clin Orthop Relat Res* 1995;321:168-172.

23. Berger RA, Rubash HE, Seel MJ, Thompson WH, Crossett LS: Determining the rotational alignment of the femoral component in total knee arthroplasty using the epicondylar axis. *Clin Orthop Relat Res* 1993;286:40-47.

24. Montgomery RL, Goodman SB, Csongradi J: Late rupture of the posterior cruciate ligament after total knee replacement. *Iowa Orthop J* 1993;13:167-170.

25. Babis GC, Trousdale RT, Morrey BF: The effectiveness of isolated tibial insert exchange in revision total knee arthroplasty. *J Bone Joint Surg Am* 2002;84-A(1):64-68.

26. Brooks DH, Fehring TK, Griffin WL, Mason JB, McCoy TH: Polyethylene exchange only for prosthetic knee instability. *Clin Orthop Relat Res* 2002;405:182-188.

27. Laskin RS, O'Flynn HM: The Insall Award: Total knee replacement with posterior cruciate ligament retention in rheumatoid arthritis. Problems and complications. *Clin Orthop Relat Res* 1997;345:24-28.

28. Archibeck MJ, Berger RA, Barden RM, et al: Posterior cruciate ligament-retaining total knee arthroplasty in patients with rheumatoid arthritis. *J Bone Joint Surg Am* 2001;83(8):1231-1236.

29. Gebhard JS, Kilgus DJ: Dislocation of a posterior stabilized total knee prosthesis: A report of two cases. *Clin Orthop Relat Res* 1990;254:225-229.

30. Kocmond JH, Delp SL, Stern SH: Stability and range of motion of Insall-Burstein condylar prostheses: A computer simulation study. *J Arthroplasty* 1995;10(3):383-388.

31. Lombardi AV Jr, Mallory TH, Vaughn BK, et al: Dislocation following primary posterior-stabilized total knee arthroplasty. *J Arthroplasty* 1993;8(6):633-639.

32. Sharkey PF, Hozack WJ, Booth RE Jr, Balderston RA, Rothman RH: Posterior dislocation of total knee arthroplasty. *Clin Orthop Relat Res* 1992;278:128-133.

33. Galinat BJ, Vernace JV, Booth RE Jr, Rothman RH: Dislocation of the posterior stabilized total knee arthroplasty: A report of two cases. *J Arthroplasty* 1988;3(4): 363-367.

INDEX

Page numbers followed by *f* indicate figures; page numbers followed by *t* indicate tables.

A

Achilles tendon, 65–66
Achilles tendon allograft, 65, 66, 69–71, 69*f*
Allograft-implant composites (AICs), 94, 96–97, 97*f*
Allografts
    Achilles tendon, 65, 66, 69–71, 69*f*
    morcellized bone, 56
    structural, 9, 57, 59
American College of Cardiology/American Heart
        Association (ACC/AHA), perioperative cardiac
        assessment guidelines of, 14
Anderson Orthopaedic Research Institute (AORI) bone
        defect classification system, 14, 49, 50*t*, 51, 52, 54, 58
Anterior synovectomy, 19, 20*f*, 26
Antibiotics
    choice of, 78–79
    postoperative, 85
    preoperative, 52, 93
    prophylactic, 43–44, 93
Aseptic loosening, 11, 30, 33
Aspiration
    for microbiologic culture, 3–4, 78
    serial, 78
Axial instability, 103, 104–106, 105*f*, 105*t*,106*f*

B

Bacterial shedding, 44
"Banana peel" exposure, 6
Body exhaust suits, 45
Bone loss
    classification of, 49, 50*t*, 51
    complications in, 59
    femoral implant removal and, 7*f*
    postoperative management, 59
    preoperative evaluation and, 51–52
    surgical technique and, 5, 7, 52–59
        cement in, 54–55
        composite allograft and custom prostheses, 59
        impaction grafting, 56–57
        metal augments, 5*f*, 55–56
        metaphyseal sleeves, 57–58, 57*f*
        morcellized allograft, 56
        porous metal cones, 58–59, 58*f*
        structural allograft, 57
Bone scintigraphy, 1, 14

C

Cement, bone loss and, 54–55
Charcot arthropathy, 11, 25
Cierny-Mader classification of osteomyelitis, 41, 42*t*
Complex regional pain syndrome, 4
Complications, following revision total knee arthro-
        plasty, 85–86
Component malrotation, 98
Composite allograft and custom prostheses, bone loss
        and, 59
Condylar fractures, 90
Constraint
    anterior and posterior cruciate ligament-substituting
        implants, 33
    in complex instability, 35
    in complex primary total knee arthroplasty, 34–35
    defined, 29
    in intraoperative MCL injury, 35
    level of
        PCL-retaining implants, 32
        PCL-substituting implants, 32–33, 33*t*
    mobile-bearing implants, 33
    in patients with patellectomy, 35
    in patients with rheumatoid arthritis, 35
    rotating-hinge implants, 34, 34*f*
    in severe valgus deformity with intact collateral liga-
        ments, 35

in severe varus deformity with intact collateral ligaments, 35
types of, 30, 31t
VVC implants, 33
Continuous passive motion devices, 8
Coonse-Adams variant of the V-Y quadricepsplasty turndown, 23
Coronal plane stability, 12
Corticosteroids, 42
C-reactive protein (CRP) level, 1, 4, 14, 51, 78
CRP. *See* C-reactive protein level.

D

Débridement in bone loss management, 57
Deep vein thrombosis, 8
Diabetes mellitus, 42

E

Ehler-Danlos syndrome, 104
Epicondylar axis, 7
Erythrocyte sedimentation rate (ESR), 1, 4, 14, 78
ESR. *See* Erythrocyte sedimentation rate.
Exposure for revision total knee arthroplasty
medial parapatellar approach, 18–19, 20–21f, 22
quadriceps snip, 22–23, 22f
skin incision, 17–18, 18f, 19f
tibial tubercle osteotomy, 24–26, 24f, 25f
V-Y quadricepsplasty turndown in, 23–24, 23f
Extensor lag, 12
Extensor mechanism disruption after total knee arthroplasty
avulsion from the tibial tubercle, 70–71, 71f, 72f
classification, 64, 64t
clinical findings, 64
etiology, 63–64
imaging, 64–65
patellar fracture, 71–72, 73f, 74f
postoperative management, 72, 74–75
preoperative preparation and surgical approach, 67, 67f
repair of patellar tendon disruption, 68–70, 68f, 69f
treatment of, 65–67

F

Femoral component
malrotation of, 109
removal, bone loss after, 7f
size of, 32
Femoral supracondylar periprosthetic fractures, 94–95

Flexion gap
balancing after implant removal, 7
determining, 31
Flexion instability, 103, 106–112, 108t, 109f, 110f, 111f
Fluoroscopic evaluation, 1, 4

G

Gait examination, 3
Gap balancing errors, 108
Gap kinematics, influence of, on stability extension gap, 30–31
Global instability, 103, 112
Goniometer, 12

H

Hematogenous seeding, 11
Hinged implants, 32
Human immunodeficiency virus (HIV), 43
Hyperextension instability, 103

I

Imaging
in extensor mechanism rupture, 64–65
in periprosthetic patellar fractures, 65
in preoperative planning, 12–14, 13f
Immunocompromised patients, risk of complications for, 43
Impaction grafting, 9, 56–57, 59
Impingement, 31
Implants
anterior and posterior cruciate ligament–substituting, 33
factors that influence choice of, 36
hinged, 32
mobile-bearing, 33
PCL-retaining, 32
PCL-substituting, 32–33, 33t
removal of, 6–7
rotating-hinge, 34, 34f
VVC, 29, 31t, 33, 36
Infections. *See also* Periprosthetic knee infections
periprosthetic knee, 14, 41–46
diagnosis of, 41
host factors in, 41–43, 42t
operating room environment in, 44–46, 45f
prophylactic antibiotics for, 43–44
revision total knee arthroplasty for, 77–86
clinical results, 85
complications in, 85–86

diagnosis of, 78–79, 78f
indications for two-stage, 77–78
postoperative care, 85
surgical pearls, 83–85
surgical technique for, 79
first stage, 79
second stage, 80–83
after total joint arthroplasty, 9, 41
Insall-Burstein prosthesis, 111
Instability
cause for primary TKA failure, 1
reason for revision total knee arthroplasty, 29–30
axial, 104–106, 105f, 105t, 106f
diagnosis of, 103–104
flexion, 106–112, 108t, 109f, 110f, 111f
global, 112
recurvatum (hyperextension) after, 106, 107f
Intraoperative culture, reliability in diagnosing infection, 78
Intraoperative MCL injury, 35

J

Joint-line height, assessment of, 13

K

Kinematic rotating-hinge knee implant, 100
Knee aspiration for microbiologic culture, 78
Knee buckling, 11
Knee Society pain score, 9

L

Laboratory tests
CRP level, 1, 4, 14, 51, 78
in determining reason for failure of total knee arthroplasty, 3–4
ESR, 1, 4, 14, 78
in preoperative planning, 14
WBC, 1, 78
Laminar airflow rooms, 45–46, 45f
Lateral gutter, débridement of, 71
Lateral parapatellar approach, 22
Lateral release, 63, 71
Ligament reconstruction, 36
Linked rotating-hinge implants, 106

M

Malnutrition, diagnosis of, 14
Malrotation, 51
Maltracking, patellar, 1, 3, 12, 63
Manipulation under anesthesia (MUA), 74–75
Mayo Clinic classification of periprosthetic patellar fractures, 64, 64t
MCL. *See* Medial collateral ligament.
Medial capsular approach, 22
Medial collateral ligament (MCL)
allograft reconstruction of, 36
attenuation, 35
avulsion of, 104
repair or reconstruction, 36
Medial gastrocnemius flap, 65
Medial parapatellar arthrotomy, 18–19, 20–21f, 22, 93
Meniscectomy, 18
Metal augments, bone loss and, 55–56
Metallosis, 30
Metal sensitivity testing, 4
Metaphyseal sleeves, bone loss and, 57–58, 57f
Midvastus approach, 18

N

Non–weight-bearing ambulation, 74
Nutritional status
assessment of, 14
impact on the risk of postoperative complications, 42

O

Obesity and risk of postoperative infection, 43
Operating room environment in periprosthetic knee infections, 44–46, 45f
Osteolysis, 4, 11, 30, 90
Osteomyelitis, Cierny-Mader classification of, 41, 42t
Osteonecrosis, 9
Osteoporosis, 90, 92
Osteosynthesis, 91, 92
Osteolytic defects, 92

P

Parapatellar arthrotomy, 52–53
Patella-post impingement, 31
Patellar clunk syndrome, 3
Patellar eversion, 6

Patellar fractures
    asymptomatic nondisplaced, 63
    etiologies of, 64
    periprosthetic, 63, 64, 64*t*, 65
    repair of, 71–72, 73*f*, 74*f*
    types, 66–67
Patellar maltracking, 1, 3, 12, 63
Patellar resurfacing, 83
Patellar tendon rupture
    physical examination for, 64
    repair of, 68–70, 68*f*, 69*f*
    treatment of, 65–66
Patellar tracking, 12
Patellar turndown, 23
Patellectomy, 17, 35
Patellofemoral implants, 14
PCL. *See* Posterior cruciate ligament.
Periprosthetic fractures
    bone defects and, 94
    classification of, 90, 91*t*
    early postoperative, 89–90
    femoral supracondylar, 94–95, 95*f*
    indications for revision total knee arthroplasty
            for, 91–92, 91*f*, 92*f*
    late postoperative, 90
    postoperative regimen in, 98
    preoperative evaluation in, 92–93, 93*f*
    results in, 98–100
    risk factors, 89–90
    surgical technique in, 93
        allograft-implant composite technique, 96–97, 97*f*
        exposure and component removal, 93–94
        general principles, 94
        pitfalls in, 97–98, 99*f*
        tibial fractures, 95–96
Periprosthetic knee infections
    diagnosis of, 14, 41
    host factors in, 41–43, 42*t*
    operating room environment in, 44–46, 45*f*
    prophylactic antibiotics for, 43–44
Periprosthetic patellar fractures
    diagnosis, 64
    following TKA, 63
    imaging for, 65
    Mayo Clinic classification, 64, 64*t*
Perivascular lymphocyte infiltration, 4
Physical examination
    in determining reason for failure of total knee arthro-
            plasty, 3, 4*f*, 5*f*
    in preoperative planning, 12, 13*f*
Polyethylene wear, 109–110
Porous metal cones, use of in bone loss and, 58–59, 58*f*

Posterior cruciate ligament (PCL)
    -retaining implants, 32
    rupture, 103
    -substituting implants, 32–33, 33*t*
Postoperative care
    bone loss and, 59
    for extensor mechanism disruption, 72, 74–75
    general protocol, 8–9
    for periprosthetic fractures, 98
    for two-stage revision, 85
Preoperative evaluation and planning, 5, 11–15
    antibiotics in, 52
    bone loss and, 51–52
    exposure in, 17
    for extensor mechanism disruption, 67, 67*f*
    history in, 11–12
    imaging studies in, 12–14, 13*f*
    laboratory analysis in, 14
    physical examination in, 12, 13*f*
    for revision total knee arthroplasty for periprosthetic
            fractures, 92–93, 93*f*
Primary total knee arthroplasty
    complex, 34–35
    incidence, 89
Prophylactic antibiotics, 43–44
Prosthesis, 29–37. *See also* Constraint
    Insall-Burstein, 111
    types of, 31*t*
Pulsatile lavage of the knee, 57, 81–82

Q

Quadricepsplasty, 19, 21*f*
Quadriceps snip, 6, 9, 22–23, 22*f*, 26, 30, 63, 93
Quadriceps strengthening, 98
Quadriceps tear, 64
Quadriceps tendon rupture
    clinical findings, 64
    treatment of, 65
Quadriceps turndown (quadricepsplasty), 6, 21*f*, 22–24, 23*f*

R

Range of motion
    assessment of, 3
    exercises for, 89
    in preoperative planning, 12
    in unstable knee, 104
Recurvatum, 103, 106, 107*f*
Rheumatoid arthritis, 26, 35, 42, 104, 110

S

Semitendinosus autograft, 65
Skin incision, in exposure for revision total knee arthroplasty, 17–18, 18f, 19f
Spacers, use of antibiotic-impregnated, in treating infection, 79–80, 80f, 81f, 82f
S-ROM mobile-bearing hinge total knee replacement, 100
Stability
    sagittal plane, 12
    technical aspects of, in revision total knee arthroplasty, 30–32
Stability extension gap, influence of gap kinematics on, 30–31
Standing alignment, testing, 3
Staphylococcus aureus, 44, 85
Staphylococcus epidermidis, 44, 85
Structural allografts, 9, 57, 59
Subcutaneous flaps, 18
Subperiosteal dissection, 19
Subvastus approach, 18
Surgical techniques
    allograft-implant composite, 96–97, 97f
    impaction grafting, 56–57
    metal augments, 55–56
    metaphyseal sleeves, 57–58, 57f
    morcellized bone allograft, 56
    for patellar fractures, 71–72, 73f, 74f
    for patellar tendon disruption, 68–70, 68f, 69f
    for periprosthetic fractures, 93–98, 95f, 97f
    porous metal cones, 58–59, 58f
    structural allograft, 57
    for tibial tubercle avulsion, 70–72, 71f
    in two-stage revision, 79–83, 80f, 81f, 82f

T

Tibial component, choosing size of, 31
Tibial periprosthetic fractures, 95–96

Tibial slope, 31
Tibial tubercle
    avulsion, 70–71, 71f, 72f
    fractures, 98
    osteotomy, 6, 9, 22, 24–26, 24f, 25f, 83, 94
Tibiofemoral dislocation, 107
TKA. *See* Total knee arthroplasty.
Total joint arthroplasty, 41
    complications after, 41
    infection after, 9
Total knee arthroplasty (TKA), primary
    long-term success of, 103
    number performed in United States, 1, 89
Transepicondylar axis, 58

U

Ultraviolet lighting to reduce surgical infection, 46
University of Pennsylvania classification of bone loss, 49

V

Varus-valgus constraint (VVC), 29, 31t, 33, 36
Varus-valgus tilt, 33
VVC. *See* Varus-valgus constraint.
V-Y quadricepsplasty turndown, 22, 23–24, 23f

W

WBC. *See* White blood cell count.
White blood cell (WBC) count, 1, 78
Wound healing, 42